Marrying Bipolar

The highs and lows of loving someone
with a mental illness

T0097634

Marrying Bipolar

The highs and lows of loving someone
with a mental illness

Natasha David

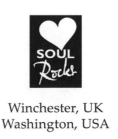

Winchester, UK
Washington, USA

First published by Soul Rocks Books, 2016
Soul Rocks Books is an imprint of John Hunt Publishing Ltd., Laurel House, Station Approach,
Alresford, Hants, SO24 9JH, UK
office1@jhpbooks.net
www.johnhuntpublishing.com
www.soulrocks-books.com

For distributor details and how to order please visit the 'Ordering' section on our website.

ISBN: 978 1 78099 584 7
Library of Congress Control Number: 2015954280

Design: Lee Nash

Printed and bound by CPI Group (UK) Ltd, Croydon, CR0 4YY, UK

We operate a distinctive and ethical publishing philosophy in all
areas of our business, from our global network of authors to
production and worldwide distribution.

This book is dedicated to my family and friends for their unfailing love and support. To Julie-Anne, my sister-in-arms. To Ian, who inspires me to pursue my best self. To Angela, who showed me what self-belief can accomplish. To Lyn, who encouraged me to write for myself.
And to Kevin, ultimately my greatest teacher.

Prologue

The Inspiration

Writing about a personal relationship is hard, made even harder in this case. The decision to do so was not made lightly. I had to overcome my natural unwillingness to look at my life during this period; my own guilt and self-doubt are contributing factors to feeling blamed for the eventual demise of my husband to suicide. I blamed myself for the inability to encourage him enough to seek treatment for what was, looking back, an obvious mental illness that was untreated far too long.

My motivations for writing this book are threefold. Firstly, in doing so, I am finally tackling head-on some major life events that happened to me and my late husband, some of which have never been disclosed outside our marriage.

Secondly, if people suffering from a mental illness feel invisible in society, their carers go even more unnoticed; usually they are the ones who cheerfully paint their faces with a smile and continue being strong, the rock of their relationships, until their strength gives out. The thought that someone, somewhere, might benefit from reading what we went through and feeling that much less alone because of it, is a driving factor for me to open up a very difficult chapter of my life.

Finally, I still hold a special place in my heart for my late husband who in many ways was a very beautiful person trapped by his past and an illness he didn't want to accept, who believed his fragility was something to deny. This is his story, and he deserves to have it told by someone who was the closest to him for the last decade of his life.

As this person, I feel privileged to have heard his stories, his version of events growing up, his attitudes and outlooks, what he went through, all those wonderful, funny, sad, tragic, mishmash of events that contributed to his makeup and life. I had an up-close and personal view of someone who battled with, and lost to, a mental illness.

It is also a daunting task because mental illness is still such a taboo subject, despite progress being made since my husband was first treated for a psychotic episode. People who are afflicted by it, live with it, love people who struggle with it, are still made to feel ashamed by both society's attitudes and also a health system that doesn't prioritise their needs to the same extent that they would if suffering a life-threatening illness such as heart disease.

People who suffer from these illnesses are made to feel doubly wrong. Both for having the illness in the first place, and then behaving in ways that they sometimes cannot control when they are in its grip, leaving many unable to engage in normal, healthy, active and full lives. My husband was one of those who struggled in this regard, and felt like a failure many times because of it.

It makes sufferers less willing and able to fight to get accurate diagnoses in the first place, access ongoing, affordable treatment, and work with professionals to access strategies to help them re-integrate as quickly as possible back into society after a critical event may have taken place. I saw this firsthand.

I hope that readers can look past the drama of the events about to unfold, and see the message underlying each chapter. Denial is never the solution to any problem, large or small. Within any relationship and especially for those who need more care and attention for any aspect of health, burying heads in the sand will only further contribute to the problem and add stress to families and social networks.

Seeking help, as early as possible, being open and honest about the pain we are all feeling at one time or another, is the answer.

Love, compassion and acceptance can all start within each and every one of us. If we can all do that within ourselves, this world will achieve the peace we'd like to experience in this generation and for generations to come.

Chapter One

The Beginning

I picked up the ringing phone at my office with a distant view of the city haze on the far horizon. It had been a busy day, typical of the hustle and bustle that went along with putting together a monthly magazine.

The voice on the other side of the line was instantly recognisable, although distant and halting.

"I'm calling to say goodbye."

The words sent a chill through my spine.

"What do you mean – 'goodbye'?"

Silence on the other end of the phone, but I could hear quiet sobbing. I knew this man, or boy as he still was in many ways, fresh out of his teens. I had discovered his age not long after we had met. I was twenty-three. He was nineteen. "NO WAY!" I said, in utter disbelief. He seemed much older than that, both in looks and demeanour. I made him take out his licence to prove it, and he obeyed, laughing, his eyes dancing in the charming way he had when he was having mischievous fun at my expense. I gave him back the licence saying "Great. I'm a cradle snatcher." Laughing, but shaking my head at the thought I was actually dating a teenager.

"I'm on the rooftop of the Madison Hotel."

My heartbeat rising rapidly now, panic setting in, "What are you doing there?"

"I'm going to jump."

By now, I was grabbing my things, stuffing them into my bag in utter panic, wanting to keep him on the phone, talking to him, making sure he was not going to do this terrible, stupid thing, seemingly out of the blue.

I can't recall the rest of that conversation verbatim, but he had

1

been calling his family and giving them the same message, I could hear the frantic beeps on his end of the line, of them trying to get through to him as well, so I instructed him to do absolutely nothing until I got there, hoping that would be enough, and hung up.

Back then, I didn't own a mobile phone, something that would be unthinkable in today's age. The thirteen-minute train ride to the city was the longest I have ever had to endure, terrified out of my wits as to what I might find, or not find, on the top of that hotel when I got there.

* * *

So, who was this man? And how did we get to this point?

It all began six months earlier at a party of a mutual friend. It was September 1996, the year following my graduation from university. I had been drifting a bit that year, not really knowing what I wanted to do with my degree, wanting to travel but not having the money to do it. Wanting to study overseas in France, but not getting the marks in my French language course to pass the strict entry requirements to their universities, and biding my time seeing "what came next". I had recently landed the job at a major Business-to-Business magazine company.

I hadn't been dating, I was despairing that I'd ever really meet anybody that understood me and my particular quirks, and resigned to the fact that the guys I liked didn't seem to like me, or vice versa!

The party was on a Sunday evening, as the crowd all worked in hospitality, making Monday the start of their weekend. I was almost ready to take my leave, in preparation for an early start to my working week, when he walked through the door.

"JOHN!" everyone cried out on spotting his happy, beaming face, and everyone lined up to be bear-hugged by this magnetic person.

I lined up behind everyone else.

Flinging out my arms for a hug, I echoed the cry "John!" with a smile, and he reciprocated with a "HELLLOOOO!" I received a massive bear hug, followed by: "Who the hell are you?"

In that instant, I ditched any idea of going home at a reasonable hour, and stayed out with John until 5 a.m. at the seedy suburb of Kings Cross, going from pub to club, talking non-stop and laughing in the same measures. I recall my exact thoughts that night, *I don't care how this man will fit into my life, but I want him in it.*

It seemed he felt the same, and we had the perfect opportunity to exchange numbers when he explained he was looking for a place to stay. It just so happened there was a place at the boarding house where I lived, a fact I eagerly disclosed. He called the next day. "Do you know who this is?"

He needn't have asked.

Moving in a week later, we spent about a month hanging out at "Melrose Place" as my friends and I that lived there dubbed our inner-city block of boarding rooms with its outdoor shared laundry and metal fire escape which served as both a place to meet and gossip, as well as a place to sit silently and admire the city lights. The building was populated by our youthful shenanigans and our habit of dropping around each other's tiny flats at all hours of the day or night.

He was handsome, light-hearted and fun to be around; the embodiment of a youthful Adonis. He would often appear in the hallway of our shared floor at the boarding house on his way to the shared bathroom wearing merely a towel around his waist, leaving me and my friend swooning in his wake. We grew to enjoy each other's company so much that it almost killed me not to know whether he felt the same way.

I remember the exact moment it happened. We went out to see a movie at the Dendy, Martin Place. The film was *Beautiful Thing,* and to this day it holds a special memory for me, such a sweet film about falling in love with unexpected people and under unusual circumstances. I guess that set the scene to fall in love.

We walked back to the bus stop on George Street, and as we did he reached for my hand, and entwined my fingers in his. As we waited for the bus in comfortable silence, he enveloped me in an embrace, very different from one of his bear hugs, and I recall the scent of his skin underneath his hooded jacket. He was like that. Sweet and endlessly affectionate.

After that day, we were virtually inseparable. Friends loved being in our company, because of the fun-loving nature of the relationship, our sociability and our endless rounds of joking around, easy-going natures and obvious ease in each other's company. We were the golden couple.

My best friend interviewed me as part of her Film and Television graduation project, which interviewed a variety of women of different ages about love. I willingly participated, answering quite honestly, "Love is about giving yourself to the other person, completely, wanting what is best for them, wanting only that they are happy. It's about sacrificing everything for their happiness."

And I honestly believed it.

I had not experienced romantic love before, and now that I had found it, I wasn't letting it go. I knew he was young. I knew he was estranged from his family for reasons he didn't seem to want to divulge at that stage, and I knew that he lived a party lifestyle, going to endless clubs, attending notorious dance parties on the Sydney clubbing scene of the late 90s. I knew he was taking recreational drugs, and living a generally unhealthy and unsustainable lifestyle. I knew his career prospects or even ambitions were not lofty at that stage. For others looking on at the relationship, with me as a well-educated, well-travelled and ambitious hard-working career woman, it might have seemed like an odd pairing.

What did I care what other people, even family and friends, thought about us? I didn't. Stubborn, I was.

* * *

Since the day I was born I exhibited an independent streak. Determined to do it "by myself", in every situation.

Family legend has a few stories that illustrate my fierce independence and unwillingness to ask for any help. At age four, I took it upon myself to walk a little friend home, across the busy street with trucks and lorries that hurtled past. "Don't worry," I told my mother when I was collected from my friend's house following what I can only assume was a frantic call from my mother to hers, "the cars stopped for us."

I was told I was not allowed to cross the road by myself until I was six. I had to be given specific goals, or I'd ignore their claims that "you can't do that" altogether. This trait has followed me well into adulthood, and exists to this day.

Another time, I instructed my mother not to accompany me on the bus only days after starting kindergarten, stating, "I can do it myself," only to get off the bus one stop early, becoming extremely disoriented and getting lost. I can still feel the sting of disappointment with myself when the lovely lady whose door I knocked on called my mother to come and walk me home. Absolutely ashamed of letting myself down, and in front of others as well. To me, being vulnerable or admitting I can't do something is like a little death of a part of myself.

Not only independent, but I 'knew it all'. Add to that a liberal dose of being a 'Susie McFixit', always lending a hand to others with their problems, probably in a subconscious attempt to avoid looking at my own. And stubborn? There was a reason my parents often called me 'Mary Mary, quite contrary' after the little girl of the nursery rhyme whose garden grew with silver bells and cockle shells and pretty maids all in a row.

At the time I met John, I had been living out of the family home for four years, supporting myself by working two jobs in the family business and a local Italian restaurant, paying my way through university and graduating free and clear from debt, all too ready and willing to start a responsible life of career-building and setting down roots in Sydney, rather than following my underlying travel itch, something that still goes fairly unscratched, even to this day. Looking at it objectively, one might say I was ripe for the picking to get deeply involved in a co-dependent relationship with someone who was very loving, yet incapable of a true partnership without substantial propping up on many levels.

However, when I look at my next few relationships following John, I see so many of the same patterns emerging that it would be unjust for me to lay the fault of our relationship becoming what it was at the feet of his illness without accepting my part as well.

Looking back on those early months, I had absolutely no idea of the tsunami about to hit me. The first time John said "I love you" was at the graduation of my best friend, the one with the film about Love, which was held ironically enough at the former mental hospital at Balmain. It came out as an outburst, followed by him running around on the lawns outside the grand buildings, arms outstretched like a plane, yelling "I love you, I love you, I love you" while I laughed.

Research has shown that the initial stages of falling in love show the same pattern of brain activity as mental impairment. In other words, our judgement is impaired, and temporary insanity sets in. So, our temporary insanity set in on the site of a former insane asylum.

Our courtship was full of incredibly sweet tales, in the beginning. He was incredibly romantic, and made plans that belied his meagre paycheque, and made me feel like a princess. I recall being taken on the Manly ferry, told to "wait and see" what he had in store (something that I could never do, impatience was a strong point of mine!)

He had organised with a local deli to prepare the most delicious feast I had ever seen. Working in his family's deli for many years, he knew to order the most exotic, delicious tasty treats for this very Aussie girl who had been brought up on meat-and-three-veg at home. I had already been instructed in the finer points of luxury lifestyle by an extended family with tendencies towards "only the very best", and was eagerly anxious to further this experimentation in my new relationship.

We laid out our spread of fresh bread, variety of cheeses, exotic fruits, stuffed vine leaves and other antipasto delights, and fresh pastries as dessert, picnic-style underneath a shelter on Manly Beach, opposite the rolling waves, watching an electrical storm about to roll into shore. It was an evening that delighted all the senses, the smell of the ocean and storm brewing in the air, the sight of the lightning, sound of thunder, taste of our meal and an intense feeling of love, warmth and companionship within each other's conversation and company.

Those sweet early days were short-lived and much missed. Perhaps the length of time we stayed together was an attempt to recapture the earlier, happier months, before the dark cloud of illness cast its shadow across everything we did.

* * *

I jumped into the elevator of the hotel, pressed the button for the top floor and prayed that I'd be able to find the stairs leading up to the roof. I was paranoid about any staff I encountered, sure they would stop me from getting there. I don't know why I didn't ask for help, or even alert the police to the situation. Back then I believe I had an instinctive protective streak that didn't want to include anyone in our problems that extended far beyond what was reasonable.

I found the stairs, was not stopped by the staff that watched me run by them, and ran across to the hunched figure sitting in the middle of the roof.

I can't recall the contents of that conversation, I was far too distraught. I do recall his avoidance of my eyes. It was as if he'd given up on himself so completely that to acknowledge anyone's presence would have been a burden on them. He spoke about his family trying to reach him, and not wanting to respond. I could only imagine how frantic they must have been.

I was already in denial, *this can't be happening*, going through bargaining, *please save him, I'll do anything if you help me get him off this roof alive*, were the thoughts that kept me going, talking to him and trying to reach him through his pain, assuring him that, "Everything will be okay, you just need help".

He described his pain as simply not wanting to be here anymore. It was all too much, and he was sick of dealing with it. With what? People who were out to "get him" or "help him", people talking about him, and the whole world being against him.

Even now, snatches of what he had already told me about his background come back to me in snippets. Times and dates now mean nothing to me, around this time. The lost friends, the mistakes he had made, a large sum of money he had won then frittered away, vicious bullying and physical abuse suffered at the boarding school he attended for the last few years of his high-schooling years, feeling like he had made the wrong choices in life at such a young age, the pressure of conforming to expectations on him. He had already been committed once already to a hospital for treatment, and didn't want to go back to that. I assured him he didn't need to, that he could stay with me, and I would take care of him (Florence Nightingale-style). He agreed on those terms to accompany me back to the street level and we found ourselves at the Glebe Community Medical Centre where doctors and nurses spoke to us about diagnosis and treatment.

The nurse who saw John immediately said, "You poor love! No wonder you are feeling so down, your whole body is as stiff as a board!"

And it was, he was carrying so much tension and stress that every single muscle had locked up. He was prescribed a cocktail of drugs to sort out his body and mind.

We were told he was experiencing a psychotic episode that may or may not result in full-blown schizophrenia. The word struck terror into both of us. We were told that it would be at least 6 to 12 months before we would know for sure. Looking back, I now believe in that moment both of us decided that he was "not going to have it", come hell or high water. Thus began the denial.

We were told there was a community outreach program, staffed by volunteer nurses, who would visit us at home once a week to check up on his progress.

My only impression of access to mental health care and treatment at a time neither he nor I could afford private doctors or psychologists or psychiatrists was that the frontline staff were doing their best with a very stretched budget and resources, but the overall effectiveness was woefully inadequate. We only had access to emergency-room and community-based care. Neither of which were personalised with continuity of care (you took a number and were seen by the next available doctor or nurse) nor deep enough to get to the core issues of why we were facing this. At no time were we referred to specialist care, owing to the inability to pay the expensive costs of treatment.

Suicide watch became my full-time job the following year.

Chapter Two

The "Episode"

Even now, that year we battled with the Episode seems so surreal to me. I can't put my finger on dates, the events get all mixed up and the thread of time unravels. All I can visualise is a big ball of twine with knobbly bits that signify the outstanding events in my memory, so if the following recounting sometimes does not seem to make sense, it is because a lot of the individual events are either mixed in together, or timeframes are condensed or elongated.

My normally photographic memory for names, events, dates and information in general has been completely wiped for this period of my life. I was recently asked whether I recall John being in hospital for part of that year. I do not recall that at all. Apparently I visited several times and met his family there as well, which I also do not remember.

In fact, I don't recall many mundane details about that year. I was still holding down a full-time job, but I have few memories of that either. The year was 1997, and that was the year this very large company moved offices, a huge move that would have taken a lot of logistics to happen. It doesn't register so much as a blip on my radar.

After much reading into post-traumatic stress disorder (PTSD) I later learned that this is what happens when someone is exposed to trauma, the brain finds ways to cope with the overload of processing it does in reaction to stress, or it simply represses information it can't cope with. It was like my brain had undergone a CTL+ALT+DLT command, and being exposed to a series of events that did not make sense, found a way to rationalise it all away or bury a lot of it altogether.

All of a sudden, all I knew was that I was in a partnership that was more nursemaid-patient than girlfriend-boyfriend. And it seemed totally and completely normal to me. Isn't that what everyone goes through? Trial by fire, to ensure their love is pure? Real? Unconditional?

As I mentioned before, I already had quite a few traits that lent themselves to being a willing participant in a co-dependent relationship. Perhaps now is a good time to explore those further.

From a very young age I displayed unusual powers of perception and mediation when it came to familial relationships. Quite often, I'd be asked to intercede on behalf of my parents to "speak to one of the other kids" about their schoolwork, their attitudes, behaviour. Quite often, I would also see an issue in communication between my parents or brothers and sister, and naturally intervene to "help them" sort it out. I could always see both sides of the equation, and had a natural talent in bringing both parties to the middle ground, or at least each other's points of view.

I honestly don't recall it being forced on me. I just had a natural inclination to help. Or to meddle. Two sides of the same coin, separated by intention.

The community nurses that attended the first few difficult months were an absolute godsend. So kind, compassionate, and despite being stretched for time and resources, always managed a cheerful disposition and caring nature. They would call us as well as visit us at home. It was such a blessing to have that, but again the length of time was limited. We had home visits for some eight weeks, and then they stopped.

When they visited, they would sit with us at my old, run-down laminate kitchen table on the third floor of the boarding house, overlooking Sydney's city skyline. The nurses would ask John how he had been feeling, how he was reacting to the medication, and would often defer to me as to diet (often poor), exercise (virtually non-existent) and signs of improvement (slow to materialise).

All the while, I was still holding down my full-time job, trying to maintain some semblance of normality. The day following the 'rooftop incident' my manager sat me down and asked me, "Are you sure this isn't manipulative behaviour?" My response, "No." Then he asked, with an undercurrent of warning that I chose not to heed, "Are you sure this is the right man for you?"

I ploughed on full-steam ahead into a relationship that I had very little knowledge of, or time to decide whether we were well-suited before the stakes were raised this high. A part of me wonders whether my natural love of drama, and the thrill of having such a big project to work on were major factors in my instant dismissal of these kinds of well-intended warnings. Why did I choose not to disengage from a relationship, remaining as friends to assist, but moving on to a healthier relationship for myself? I will never know, and perhaps my calling was to go through what I was about to go through to become the person I am today. No one can ever speculate the "what ifs" and as they say, hindsight is 20-20. I hadn't even paused to get my glasses on at this stage. Unless they were rose-tinted, I was good at grabbing that pair!

John was obviously unfit to continue work, and went on disability benefits, a pittance that did nothing to enhance his self-esteem or ability to aspire to any sort of lifestyle that he had previously been used to. Not a lavish lifestyle, but it had been above the poverty line. Going to Centrelink to collect his pension was humiliating for him, as he was naturally a hard worker and very proud of being able to live away from home.

His medication caused him to put on a massive amount of weight, puffing up around his face, and his once-chiselled six-pack buried now under a layer of belly fat. He was very depressed about this as well, losing confidence in himself and self-esteem was the hardest thing to watch. His meds also dulled his bright and sociable personality. He became distant, moody and withdrawn from me and others.

There was a different look about him that has since been echoed by partners of other sufferers. They can, with an instant, look entirely different from the person they once were, a dark shadow literally crosses their faces, and with John I could see the change arriving with the dulling of his eyes. A lifeless stranger would suddenly be looking back at me, devoid of recognition or emotion. It was chilling.

I can understand why in the Dark Ages people who suffered from mental illnesses were often accused of being possessed by demons. If a person's consciousness is called their soul, then I can easily see those moments of transition being interpreted as the dark side of John's soul taking over his body. It was literally like watching a possession by his own demons. The side I privately referred to as Mr Hyde.

I would often come home from work to find John sitting at the kitchen table, obsessively reading the same paragraph of a book over and over again, convinced it was "talking to him", and giving him messages. He could never quite explain what those messages were, but they were always negative, about how much of a loser he was, how he would never amount to anything. My rational assurances and explanations that the book was written and published well before he was born didn't make one iota of difference to him. Neither reason nor calming tone could soothe Mr Hyde once he had awoken. He was unfortunately resident until he decided it was time to go away. The medication didn't seem to completely put him to rest.

Sometimes John would come home very late from having taken a bus but alighting many stops before home, and would insist he had to get off because the people on the bus had been "talking about him" and laughing. I would try in vain to diffuse his paranoia – "Did it occur to you that they may have just been telling funny stories and laughing about that?" Once again, rational explanations about what might have been going on completely eluded him.

One night he didn't come home at all, and I was beside myself with worry, wondering what had happened to him. He turned up in the small hours the next morning, telling me he had to climb a tree in a nearby park to "get away from the cars that were following me." What cars? The peak-hour traffic that might have been using that street to get home? I could only watch on in helplessness, to this man who was battling some incredibly hard inner demons, and losing more often than winning. It must have been exhausting for him, as much as it was for me who was caring for him full time.

I had only ever seen the world as a place where amazing things can happen. Thanks to my relatively healthy and happy upbringing, it was full of possibilities. Thanks to my education, it was full of opportunities. Thanks to my family and friends, it was full of love.

Being with John, I started to see a different world. A world through the eyes of a sufferer of mental illness. It was a very bleak place, and distressing to watch John's reaction to it. Frightening. Pursuing him. Evil. Out to get him.

From month six until the year after experiencing the extreme psychotic episode, we began to see some improvements. Enough for him to seem stable and get a job with a call-centre agency. John started to rebuild a little confidence with his independence, but we were not out of the woods just yet. We had been told of a support group for people with schizophrenia, and John went to one session. When he came back I was eager to hear how it all went.

He said, "Oh, I'm not going back, it is too depressing there and the people are all really sick. There are far worse people there than me, compared to them I'm fine."

He never went back for another session. Looking back now, I wish I had insisted on it, as the relapse into his former lifestyle was not too far off. However, this was to be a pattern perpet-uated, and encouraged by me, throughout our entire relationship. I would see an issue, explain he needed to get help or support to fix it, we would get to the point of fighting about it, eventually he would reluctantly go, usually with me shoving documents or brochures in his face, then his response would be "I'm not as bad as the others, I'm fine" and stop going. It was easier and less hassle to just give in, from a couple's point of view. From a carer point of view, it was remiss of me to not keep at it. However, he had been given the all clear at the end of that period that it had not, in fact, turned into full-blown schizophrenia, and I think we were both way too eager to believe that.

We were starting to get a semblance of normality to our lives, or at least trying to pretend we were a normal couple. This was the period during which rebuilding his ties back to his family was of utmost importance to me. I had heard his side of things, but being such a family-oriented person, I had the firmly held opinion that broken fences should be mended.

A lot of his problems, I later worked out, stemmed from moving out of his childhood home to lead a very hedonistic, party lifestyle, including drug-taking, alcohol abuse, gambling and also unhealthy partnerships in general. He had, in effect, fallen in with the wrong crowd.

By the time I met his family, it was obvious they were distressed at losing touch with John, and loved him dearly. They only wanted what was best for him, but as a young man, like so many other young men, he was merely interested in the present moment, with little thought to the future.

By the time his lifestyle caught up with him, his paranoia with people "helping" him was complete. He resented being told what to do and interpreted every single gesture of reaching out by all family members as wanting to do him harm.

Slowly, however, we were able to show him through patience and compassion that this was not the case. I credit my influence on him being the reason he was open enough to rebuilding those relationships, as I was the only one he trusted at that time. He was also running away from financial difficulties, and had incurred considerable debts and unpaid bills which he chose to ignore, leading to debt-collection agencies chasing him down and building up a bad credit record in general. This did not bode well for a stable future for us! But still, I ignored the warning signs.

His parents were always there to help him out, and yet these gestures, meant with the best of intentions, only fuelled his belief that in his parents' eyes he didn't measure up to his very smart and capable sisters who were already on their way to successful careers and lives of their own. He constantly felt he let his family down being who he was, and that he was expected to be so much more than where he was in life. He felt the pressure to lead a life that his parents could be proud of.

However, what parent doesn't want this for their children? His parents were very hard workers, who were given no handouts in life, yet through hard work and sacrifice aimed to make their children's lives better through education and opportunities they never had.

When I finally met them, they had built a comfortable yet frugal life and were now focused on watching their adult children forge careers and relationships, and were eagerly anticipating their next stage in life to be grandparents. They were excited to be leaving to a legacy of grandchildren they so longed for from all their progeny.

That first year of our courtship, both his sisters moved to the UK to pursue their careers, which left his parents as his only family support system during the interim years. That year seemed to be the end of our troubles, for a time.

Our optimism was further demonstrated by moving from the very cheap boarding-house living arrangements into a little one-bedroom workman's cottage in the inner-west of Sydney, committing to a year-long lease. The weekly rental on that place was meagre, yet stretched our budget completely, but was manageable now that John was working again.

The little half-house was bright mustard yellow on the outside, with mission-brown trim. The tiny little rooms at the front, one serving as a living room, and the other as our bedroom, had no wardrobes or storage space at all. Our clothes hung from two clothing racks. Our kitchen had no bench space, and a three-ring electric burner stove with a temperamental oven. There was inadequate lighting throughout, and no light outside. The lean-to bathroom had lino laid straight onto the dirt floor, and our only toilet was an outhouse, also with no light. We had a tiny little back garden that was overgrown with patchy grass, weeds and dirt.

But it was our first home together. All ours. We were so proud.

And, above all, it created an outward semblance of normality.

We furnished the place with furniture that was either donated or scrounged from thrift stores, or bought on next to nothing. What we lacked in interior decor we made up for with love of each other and love of filling that house with guests, visitors and parties. We threw a big house-warming party, and filled that house with amazing smells of cooking and sounds of laughter.

But it was not all beer and skittles, this move to commit myself further to this man. Medication given to sufferers of a mental illness wreaks a number of side effects. The obvious one is weight gain, which can lead to poor self-esteem and lack of energy to do anything. Another is the dulling of the person's real personality, so someone who is normally bubbly, sociable and likes doing things, will have little interest or energy to do things that once gave them pleasure or fun. As if that wasn't enough to impair a relationship, the meds also had the side effect of killing all traces of a normal libido. Something that would have far-reaching impact on our entire time together and our ability to build any normality of intimacy as a couple.

Chapter Three

The Background

What causes mental illness in adults?

From what I have read, and I did read extensively and obsessively after it all fell apart, is that the causes are mostly complex and largely unknown. I will attempt to draw my own parallels between what is known from reading scientific research to what I observed which is, of course, highly unscientific yet a layman's attempt to make some sense of how it came to be for John.

Genetics play a part. In fact, this was something drawn to my attention during our relationship, as John always expressed the desire for children "when we get married", and was anxious to ensure I felt the same way. While I love children, I have always felt ambivalent about having my own, but because of the love I felt for this man, I could not rule out that one day I might suddenly wake up and want them as badly as he did! I mention children now, because he brought my attention to the genetic predisposition of passing on mental illness. He cited research he had done himself, that there was a 36% chance that a sufferer of schizophrenia would pass that tendency on to children. However, because he was better, we quickly dismissed that fact.

I could also see how the very traditional values of the culture could also exacerbate this, so it may have been combination of both. It certainly didn't help the fact that he felt pressure to conform to taking on the role of provider, the constant references to how I would always earn more than him betrayed an attitude that the man should be the breadwinner, and I know it caused him considerable embarrassment and stress when those in our circle pointed to my success instead of his.

I felt the constant need to downplay my own successes and talents, to try to shy away from the limelight, something I find very hard to do as a natural entertainer. I would often be accused of showing off once we got to the privacy of our own home after a night of socialising, and me naturally taking centre stage or making some clever quip or remark. We once watched a French film with another couple, and my remark "I love this film" was met with a glowering comment "only because you like people knowing you speak French". It was impossible to respond to these remarks. It became virtually impossible to separate the issues in our relationship that were caused by mental instability, and those caused by incompatibility.

Disease, injury and infection can also be a trigger. Any normal upbringing of boys, indeed children in general, can include any or all of these things. However, it seemed that John had a number of childhood illnesses that could also have played a part. Certainly during early adulthood, John led a very unhealthy lifestyle, including poor nutrition, and recreational drug use, which are all linked to onset mental illness in young men aged between nineteen and thirty.

Mental characteristics have been linked to development and maintenance of mental disorders. These include the way a person thinks or perceives events – John was always misinter-preting events to be far worse or more personalised than they actually were. Overall personality and coping style plays a part. John was always referring to learning from my "ability to cope with stress", something I thought little of until I realised he didn't cope with it at all. There are also links to an individual's protective factors, or "positive illusions" such as optimism, personal control, and overall meaning of life. These factors seemed present only in their extremes with John. When he was "up", he was overly positive, to the extent of poor decision-making and risk-taking. My personality is also risk-seeking, so I didn't think too much of this at the time. In hindsight, however, I can link these extreme swings from positive to negative to be in line with behaviours exhibited with bipolar, something that later on a range of psychologists and other specialists would identify as the possible illness John suffered from.

Life events, emotional stress and relationships are another factor. These are things that John had been dealt in spades. He often spoke of tyrannical bullying he endured at a boarding school where he was educated for the final years of his school years. The physical abuse culminated in his being held by his arms and given a severe beating by every single senior boy of that school. For what? Defending his best friend, who was also being bullied relentlessly. The ringleaders made his best friend start the proceedings, and John often recounted the haunted look his friend gave him which never left his memory. After the incident he ran away for three days and begged to be allowed to leave the school.

He also had suffered emotional stress from poor decisions as a young man. For example, crashing the family car into a service station, and covering up the outcome by representing himself in court, negotiating with the owners to pay for the damage, losing his licence and subsequently having to move out of his parents' semi-rural home and into the city where he stood a better chance of getting work. I believe the emotional toll on John from this one episode itself was the cause of most of the later poor decisions, and exposed him to a lifestyle he may not have otherwise sought out.

One more important piece of background information was the gambling addiction that started when he won a significant jackpot on a poker machine, which led to him quitting his job, and partying it up for three months, gaining many friends and generally being the life and soul of the party set. It also set the scene for hooking him on the illusion of a "get rich quick" mentality, rather than building something from the ground up and maintaining it through hard work and perseverance. He would continue to chase that win for the rest of his life.

But was the mental illness the cause or was it the outcome of all of these events that occurred well before I even met John. Was he already earmarked for a hard life, his gentle and loving nature to be sacrificed to mental pain and anguish? How much of the John that I saw was his illness, and how much was it simply his personality, being unable to face issues and ignoring or running away from problems?

If he did not have to succumb to such events, would he have lived a normal life?

Chapter Four

The Early Years

"Why don't you leave me. Please go. I'm no good for you."

Cold, lifeless eyes looked at me, unrecognising and unresponsive. The dark shadow had passed across his face only minutes before. We'd argued, and now he was asking me to break up with him.

It was the first time I allowed myself to breakdown. A volcano erupted from the lump rising in my throat, and I never knew tears could actually spring outwards from force of emotion. Unable to speak, gasping for air and sobbing hysterically, John was shocked out of his self-imposed prison, possibly for the first time in our relationship understanding the depth of my feelings.

But how was I actually feeling? Was it grief? Or relief? A number of thoughts ran through my head in that moment. I recount them here without judgement, and invite you to perhaps view from a relatively safe distance how the partner of someone with mental instability, who thought they were looking at the light at the end of the tunnel and then realising it was actually a train hurtling back towards them, might be feeling.

How can he do this to me again? When is it my turn to be looked after? We just signed a twelve-month lease, I can't afford this place on my own. He can't afford this place on his own. How can we split up now, we've just gone through the worst. Haven't we? Oh God, we haven't, have we. I don't want to go through that again. But I don't want to lose him either. What if I just walked away. Maybe it would be better. I'm so tired of this. Is there anyone else out there for me? Would they make me feel the way he does? How can I love anyone else? I just want things to go back to the way they were.

All these thoughts flicked through my mind, until I clutched at the one emotion that felt comfortable to me. Love.

"I'm not going to leave you."

We didn't break up that day. And he never brought it up again, until the end, writing "maybe Natasha should have left me when I asked her to. I wouldn't have been happy, but maybe she would have been."

* * *

It wasn't all bad, though. Those early years also had some amazingly good times. However, looking back on them, many happy memories are from times I spent travelling on my own. And coming back to my man when I'd had a break.

That year I travelled to New Zealand with my best friend from university. John didn't like that idea much, as he couldn't afford to come with us. We had tried to encourage him to save alongside us, scraping together our meagre funds to buy an all-inclusive ski package to Queenstown. I had hoped this enforced savings plan would encourage John to start being a little more fiscally responsible. He really wanted to, but he didn't do it. His love of the good life was back again, and he would go out with his workmates after his door-to-door sales job, and sometimes blow his entire weekly paycheque on beers or pokies. He loved to shout his friends drinks. He smoked. And he was always the last man standing. A night out could easily cost him hundreds of dollars. I loved him for his generosity of spirit, but I wished it came with a regulator switch.

So, I went on the trip and endured the very frequent phone calls from John who called morning, noon and night. He was naturally very cautious about his girlfriend sharing a room (but not a bed) with a male friend. We laughed at the time, as our friendship was and always has been platonic. But John was incredibly jealous of any male friend in our social circle as many were openly complimentary about me. He harboured a jealous streak and his paranoia eventually extended to my natural bubbliness and affectionate warmth towards our friends.

I had also always been a keen motorbike lover. Up to that point I didn't have any spare cash to purchase any kind of vehicle of my own, although by that stage I'd already lent John the money to purchase his first car, a Mitsubishi Colt which cost as much to run and repair as it had to purchase.

I bought my first motorbike. A little Honda CB250, which became another escape. I might not have acknowledged it consciously back then, and would never have admitted it to John even if I had, but I needed an escape route. A safety valve, even. The first long trip I did was with a women's motorbike group from university, who rode with me nestled within their humming beasts all purring with 500cc engines and above, my little 250cc Honda puttering all the way up the NSW coastline to Valla Beach. Staying overnight in cabins with this boisterous, happy, friendly bunch was the happiest time I can recall from that year. Riding back home the next day was exhausting, but oh so satisfying!

Being welcomed with a smile by John when I got home was even better, having been given a reprieve from each other's patterns for days was a good thing.

I also have some great memories from that period. We started our Sunday Big Breakfast ritual in that house. Every single Sunday, without fail, we'd walk down to the local shops to buy the papers. When we got home, I'd cook up a storm. Despite only having three electric burners and limited bench space, I managed to consistently turn out poached eggs, toast, bacon, roast tomatoes, mushrooms, plunger coffee and orange juice, all served on our rickety wooden table in our tiny backyard. And every single Sunday John would beam at me when I served it all up, taking one bite of his eggs, saying "you make the best eggs." From someone who was used to doing silver service in his first career, I considered that the highest compliment.

As we ate we would complete the Sunday crosswords together. John would never fail to make me laugh hysterically at his original crossword-solution style. It was more a word associ-ation game than guessing the correct synonym to a word. And he'd completely ignore the existing letter placement. It was hilarious and he totally played up to it, delighting in my mirth.

We shared many happy moments in that house together, and if we didn't have the dark cloud of John's illness to deal with, there is no doubt we would have been a couple that lasted forever. However, it is the crises that seem to lodge themselves more firmly into my memory and stay there, with the pink-heart moments fading to become a background colour to our relationship. There were reasons I stayed with this man for so long, throughout the extreme periods of difficulty. Laughter and love were the two main ones. I can endure pretty much anything if those two elements are present.

* * *

One night, I came home to find John smoking a joint and erupted in fury.

"How dare you risk your state of mind again, have you got absolutely no regard for your health at all? I can't do this any longer, I'm leaving."

I called my father that night to collect me, which he did without question. Hearing his daughter sobbing on the phone in obvious distress must have been a difficult thing. He came instantly and without question. I was stony faced and quiet all the way home, unable and unwilling to illuminate why I was so furious. I didn't want to let anyone know why I was so furious with John, as it would mean admitting he was not taking his condition seriously.

It was only much later that I revealed the transgression. Something that would happen more regularly than I cared to admit.

Of course, I went back.

* * *

Why did I go back? The signs were all there, from the instability to the inability to face his demons, his illness, or even the fact that something was terribly, terribly wrong with our relationship. Why were my needs constantly being downplayed in my effort to tiptoe around Mr Hyde? Why was he happy to continue in fantasy land, where actions have no consequences and the pieces are left for other people to pick up?

Why, in other words, was this relationship continuing against all odds?

That year, the night terrors began. In the middle of the night, I would be awoken by a primal scream that would go on and on, terrified out of my mind, and cringing with embarrassment knowing that through the walls our neighbours would hear that sound.

I would confront John about those yells. What was he dreaming? He couldn't remember. Was he worried about something? He didn't know. What had happened to him in the past to provoke such terror? He refused to engage in conversation.

Not much later than the yells began, I was woken from a deep sleep by a king hit punch to my solar plexus. I sat straight up in bed, gasping for breath, winded to my core. Frightened, confused and in flight mode, I jumped straight out of bed and looked back down at John. He appeared to be awake, his eyes black and his face stone cold, looking at me with hatred.

I couldn't speak from lack of air. I couldn't move back towards the bed as I was so terrified by what had happened. Was he awake? Did he intend to do that? Did he know?

We never spoke about it.

That would happen again and again, sometimes I'd be awoken by a barrage of blows to my head, like he was fighting off an enemy that was coming at him. The blows were always scattered, heavy and out of control.

I'd later beg John to see a psychologist to help him unlock these episodes, as he claimed they were never intentional. But I was sick of bearing the brunt of his unnamed fears. I was getting tired of him pretending there was nothing wrong, and moving on like we didn't have anything to discuss. So long as we were together, that meant things were okay with him.

* * *

If you had told me I'd be in a physically abusive relationship, and stay there for years to come, I'd have always laughed and told you I'd leave at the first sign of violence. How, then, did I rationalise this one away? Well, firstly he never knew what was happening. He was either unconscious or denying he knew what had happened. He said he never remembered hitting me in his sleep.

Looking back on it now, though, if your partner was being beaten around by someone else, you'd hold that person accountable and not stop until you made sure it didn't happen again. I can see this was another denial of any alternative part of his personality, the denial of Mr Hyde. The inability or unwillingness to face something that was actually physically hurting his partner. He didn't want to face the demons, never wanted to get to the bottom of where it came from. Never mind the emotional and mental toll on my psyche in denying there was anything ever wrong.

I became one of those women who would cover it up on behalf of their partners, saying internally "he didn't mean it".

* * *

We received news that one of his sisters was to be married in the UK. I had always wanted to travel to that part of the world, eager to see the history and places of interest firsthand that were constant references from my love of reading since a very young age.

I did an immense amount of research for that trip. I was determined not to waste a single moment or miss an opportunity. I mapped out all the places I've always wanted to go, and drew up our own itinerary, without any help from travel agents. It was a labour of love and a work of art. But I was constantly belittled for it, being told "I prefer to be spontaneous". I don't think John understood or cared to understand my need to feel in control over things I could control. His need for unstructured, spontaneity had only gotten us in trouble before, so I was absolutely sticking to my guns that this was the way we would be travelling together. It caused many an argument, and a lot of silences between us, but in the end he admitted it was the trip of a lifetime.

John later admitted he thought I would leave him after the trip, something I had no intention of doing. Each year I'd think *this has to be the year it gets better* and I was honestly optimistic about that. Each year from this time onward, however, seemed to get a little worse, and things would happen that made me wonder whether I was actually on the right path at all, for myself, let alone for John.

* * *

That year also marked the beginning of my career trajectory. Something in hindsight, I can see adding to the rift in our paycheques, status and compatibility of life goals. I also started studying my MBA in Technology Management, again putting pressure on both time spent together and highlighting the difference in our goals and general abilities.

It marked the year John started taking his own life a bit more seriously. He wanted to get ahead, or even just to catch up to where I was in life. At that stage, he had done no real study, so sitting down with his parents to try to guide him to where we wanted to be, ultimately, he decided that marketing was the career for him and enrolled in a Diploma of Marketing at TAFE.

He did extremely well, applying himself to study and getting one of the highest marks in his final assignment, assisting a start-up online dating company develop their marketing plan at a time this industry was still in its infancy. John saw something valuable in the information and data these sites would go on to collect and his recommendations were taken on board and as far as I know, probably still used today.

We had both decided that year, as well, to move back home to our respective parents' abodes to save as much as we could to purchase a house together. I achieved our target savings quite easily, but John fell short. Again, it became a point of comparison he would bring up again, feeling ashamed he didn't hit the mark.

Living apart for the most part that year, helped diffuse our issues, and seeing each other on weekends gave us the impression that all our previous problems had disappeared. We were happy again, a loving couple, living normally and planning for a future together.

* * *

"Let's take a break, you've been studying too hard."

John had come into the dining room of his parents' house, my papers were strewn over the table. Hunched over my work, I looked up and saw he was carrying a picnic basket.

"Where are we going? Do I need to change?"

I was decked out to the nines in my tracksuit pants, t-shirt and hoodie and the final touch to my outfit were my ultra-comfortable, ultra-sexy knee-high Ugg boots.

"No, just come with me, it's all packed and ready."

We drove a little way up the quiet street his parents lived in, then made a right-hand turn at the roundabout. Another turn down an even quieter street and I was intrigued.

"Where are we going?"

"It's a place I used to ride my bike all the time when I was a kid. I loved coming here. You'll like it, it's really peaceful."

We parked at a dead end of the road, and John led me, carrying the picnic basket, through a thicket of bushland. Luckily he knew the way, there was no path and I couldn't see where we were heading.

Suddenly, the bush opened up to a sandy inland river. It was one of those little oases only locals would ever stumble over and know about. It was lovely. We sat down on a fallen log, and started to unpack the picnic basket. I was anxious at this stage, knowing how much work I had to do, and kept babbling about the stupidest things.

John was very quiet. In a pause in my chit chatter, he said, "You're going to marry me, aren't you?"

It was a question I'd heard a million times before, he had started asking this, almost anxiously, very early on, almost as if he needed to hear my assent before he could continue what he was doing. I thought this was just another one of those times. Sighing, I responded, "Sure I will."

I looked around, and he was holding out a box. I was gobsmacked. I could only manage to say, "You tricked me!"

He was smiling, and I accepted the box, with a rose gold band and channel set diamonds, very small, very quiet, and very much to my taste for someone who does not wear jewellery. He would later get teased about the lack of ostentation, but I didn't care.

"I guess that means we're engaged."

Possibly the least romantic thing anyone's ever said to accept a proposal. But I was honestly shocked. I also punched him in the arm for allowing me to get engaged while wearing tracksuit pants and Ugg boots, but deep down I loved that part too.

Chapter Five

The Married Years

It's one of those things, when you've been with someone long enough, and they give you an engagement ring, you simply accept that's the normal order of things. I'd always told John that marriage was not of great importance to me. It wasn't the end-point I'd ever sought from a relationship, and I could take or leave the concept altogether.

I meant it. My mother and her sisters recall me announcing as a wee young girl, "I'm never getting married and I'm never having kids." They laughed at the time, naturally, saying I'd feel differently when I grew up and fell in love. I secretly thought I knew my own mind better. And sure enough, I grew up, fell in love, and still didn't feel passionately about either situation.

But getting married was of utmost importance to John. He was a traditional family man, with deeply held views about marriage, children, and holding my hand protectively whenever we'd cross the street. Something I found both endearing and also a little smothering.

Nonetheless, I found myself engaged and hurtling towards a wedding that I increasingly found to be more of a burden than pleasure to organise. I was working flat out at this point, in an under-resourced office where I was under incredible pressure to turn out the volume of work previously done by three staff!

My mother ended up doing a lot of organising on my behalf. Initially I wanted to go overseas and get married with anyone who wanted to come with us. That would disappoint too many people, I was told, not the least of which would be my maternal grandparents. I was the apple of my grandmother's eye, so I ditched that idea.

While I harboured dreams of having a less-formal cocktail

party, where people could wear party dresses and have fun dancing the night away, I was informed that my guests would expect to sit down to a meal. I gave up and acquiesced on this point, but in my usual stubborn ways, I stood firm on opting out of the traditional bridal elements that were expected of me from both sides of the family. I opted to be married in a garden rather than a church, I didn't want to wear the veil or the garter, and I certainly wasn't throwing a bouquet. This was all commented upon on the day. It seemed that weddings were public property, and my own views should have been played down to please others.

Bridezilla I was not, taking an increasingly casual view of the whole event, instructing my bridesmaids to select their own dresses, which didn't need to match. They did find two dresses that were identical, in a grey-green hue that complemented both of them extremely well. My dress made from the cream lace curtain offcut I had found in the cast-off section of a material store. It cost a pittance. I teamed it with a slip made of gold material. It was an extremely simple dress, to suit my simple tastes.

The invitations were home-made with the help of a creative friend. I bought Australian native flowers at the markets the day before, filling the van full of blooms for a song. The bouquets were gathered into place with a simple cream ribbon, and the rest were decorations for the day.

The day dawned with rain clouds threatening to break. The wedding was meant to take place in a local rose garden. However, standing in my underwear that morning looking at the clouds looming beyond the covered pergola at my parents' home, I made a snap decision.

"We'll have the wedding here."

My brothers were quickly deployed to divert guests arriving at the rose garden to the family home. However, no one thought to inform the groom and his party! The bridal car circled the local suburbs waiting for the all-clear to arrive while someone called the groom and told them to make their diversions.

Apart from the shaky beginning to the day, another moment stands out in my mind. My nervous groom, who had been rehearsing his vows repeatedly earlier that day, mistakenly said, "I take you as my life" instead of "wife". We all had a good laugh at the mishap, but it became sadly prophetic in the end.

In the end, it was a beautiful day, and we both had a lot of fun, despite the battles fought to get there. We danced and ate, and talked to friends, and generally enjoyed the party that it was. However, the day eventually took its toll on me, and as soon as I found myself flagging in energy, wanted to get out of there as soon as possible, so we said our goodbyes and left to get into the bridal car to zoom us away to our hotel to spend our first night together as husband and wife.

* * *

We started our married life living at his childhood home. At this stage, we had not found our house, and were searching high and low for the right place within our budget. I was commuting up to three hours a day, by train. Something that took its toll both physically and mentally. However, we were both eternally grateful for the leg-up in life, as it allowed us to save further for our home.

We were destined for our future home, seeing it for the first time was a serendipitous moment. I was having lunch with two friends from my university days, and as we walked past a real estate agency in Parramatta, one of them pointed out a delightful two-bedroom semi-detached house in Mays Hills, a tiny pocket suburb between the M2 and the Great Western Highway in the western suburbs of Sydney. I fell in love with it the moment I walked through the front door, and we signed the contract that very day.

It was, as one family member described it, like a dollhouse. Larger than our first shared home, it felt like we were playing house on the next level. It was our patch of dirt, with a backyard that lent itself to the entertaining we were to do regularly.

Our little home became the focal point for our circle of friends. My best friend from university bought a bachelor pad within walking distance, and became a regular fixture at our home most weeks. He became a sounding board for many of our disagreements, always fair and equitable in his mediation of the situation, becoming indispensable in helping me unravel what was fair and what were unreasonable expectations from John. He was also very good at drawing from John his inner thoughts and feelings, another reason we had a great chance at heading off any unhealthy patterns in those early years. His wisdom and caring nature were amazing in helping John in many ways, in particular when I would be overseas for work for weeks or months at a time, dropping in to ensure John was looking after himself (usually he wasn't).

John was socialising a lot more as well at this stage. He had a group of friends to go out with, and would also often visit my brothers who would organise large poker parties. His general lifestyle was drinking a lot, smoking a lot and the occasional recreational drug here or there. I decided at this point I was not his mother, and pretty much said, "It's up to you, but if your health fails again it's not my problem."

But of course, it was.

This became a period of my life where I started to question some of our values in the relationship. John was adamant that we started thinking about having a family, particularly as a few in our group already had small children, which made him more determined.

John was amazing with children. They responded to his gentle nature and would always open up to him with their own fears and worries. I can still recall some amazing conversations he would later recount to me, and I could see he naturally related to children and helped them in many ways. I believe John was emotionally fixed in his childhood, owing to a traumatic incident which occurred to him within primary school years. However, his emotionally childlike state was frustrating for me, as much as it was a boon in his friendships with children. He could get a deeper understanding of their feelings than anyone else in our adult circles.

We would often argue about this point. My views were that children were a commitment for life, so I was not about to enter into that one lightly. He had to give me a convincing argument to make up my mind.

In the end, he convinced me. I fell pregnant, twice. I miscarried, twice. The first time I was about to go to Hong Kong to deliver a four-day consultancy project, and had to call John from the doctor's waiting room. He was devastated. I felt only relief.

I must have normalised an incredible amount of stress around that time, so much so that my body decided that carrying a child was something it simply could not do. I was the main bread-winner, with John in between jobs again, having quit his marketing job without consulting me. Something he was prone to do in a fit of pique. I was also bearing the main load of running a home, as well as treading on eggshells waiting for the next appearance of Mr Hyde or the next bout of gambling losses that drained our bank account from our carefully budgeted funds.

I was also stressed from trying to encourage us both to consistently lead a healthier lifestyle. Cooking more vegetables, which John mostly refused to eat, and avoiding pastas and heavy meals that he favoured. It was exhausting work, essentially raising a child who was a fully grown adult!

I was also running regularly with my best mate and my sister, in my efforts to slim down to become more attractive for John, who had told me on several occasions that my weight was a turn-off. He would compare me to my slimmer, attractive friends and say, "Why can't you be more like her?" I later learned that I was often complimented to John by their partners, something that he didn't take kindly to. Something I bore the brunt of. At this stage I was a healthy and attractive weight, but felt like an elephant, unable to keep my attraction within my marriage. It was amazing we fell pregnant twice!

So, was it any wonder my body simply refused to play ball, and cared for me the only way it could, by eliminating what could have been an even more catastrophic stress on my plate at a time I was already struggling with so much.

There was so much unexpressed pain being kept secret. The lies we told ourselves, and others would eventually be our undoing. This was not just confined to John and myself, it extended throughout the family. I would often see outbursts of emotion in reaction to tightly held pain that they hadn't found a healthier way to communicate and express. It could have set up the coping patterns each of them carried forward into their relationships. Was I any better, though? My reason for keeping my pain close to my chest was the shame that I couldn't fix it this time. That I would be failing in everyone else's eyes.

Chapter Six

The Good Bits

So far I have concentrated mainly on incidents, examples and events that are all focusing on Mr Hyde. I haven't really outlined or elaborated on the better parts of John's nature, and the good parts of our relationship. People may now wonder what possible reason I could have had to stay. It's too easy in hindsight to focus on the negatives and give an overall impression of someone that is very very opposite to how they were most of the time.

His friends who knew him during this period, in particular, would have a great deal of difficulty reconciling the happier outward parts of his personality to his private darker side. I think this is part of the reason why it was such a shock that the next few years saw such a rapid decline in our relationship and the ultimate decision John made, which seemed to come out of the blue for everyone but myself who had lived through the cycles of pain.

From what I have read about bipolar, the illness has a certain rhythm to it, called cycling. People can go from high-performing, happy upbeat phases, to the downswings, in either a long-term cycle or rapid cycling. John's cycles seemed to last for a few months when he would spiral into his "down" phases, leaving the rest of the time to be mainly a happy and positive experience.

There was a lot of fun, John always knew how to joke, and our conversations were peppered with laughter and jovial chit chat. Whenever I would suggest an outing, he'd be all in and then some, when he was in his "upbeat" cycle. We went camping quite regularly with friends, and you wouldn't have been able to spot any difference. He would accompany me on some of my longer motorbike trips, for Camp Quality, helping the kids with cancer have a good fun time, staying in cabins and generally being part of that side of my life.

We visited my grandparents in regional NSW quite often, often he was the instigator of those trips, as he loved their company, playing endless rounds of card games with my grandmother, then keeping Pop company in the evenings with his rounds of Johnnie Walker. My grandparents loved him dearly, and always welcomed him into their home, finding his company to be uplifting and rewarding.

He had a deep side, and we could talk for hours about things that really mattered. Life, the universe, everything. He cared deeply about people. He really listened to you and heard you. And would remember what you said, and all of a sudden he would surprise you with a little comment you had made, that he recalled and acted on months later.

His affectionate nature was always evident, and he would always kiss and hug me hello or goodbye, and we'd always try and sort out our differences before the end of the day. He was very protective of me when we were in public, making sure I was safe if we crossed the street, and in general was an absolute gentleman with females in our company, ensuring they were also comfortable and safe.

John's respect and love for my family was beyond reproach. He wanted to be part of the gang and respected my brothers and sister like they were his own. He lived in fear of letting any of my family down, partly the reason I kept so much from them so as not to damage his relationship with them. He cared about every family member he met of mine during our relationship, my vast hordes of cousins, remembering each by name, their partners and their children. He always had a good time with them and included himself in their lives and loves.

We had a contest with our "I love you"s. They would go back and forth "I love YOU more", "I love YOU more", until we fell about laughing.

Christmas was a special time for John. He would always

decorate a tree, was a great gift selector, once calling his best mate to get his shorts size because he happened to see a pair that would be perfect for him. He was a thoughtful person.

For the most part, he was universally upbeat and happy. He was always smiling, bear hugging and welcoming of everyone that came into his path, and I loved his open and generous ways. As mentioned, sometimes I wished he was a little more careful with his generosity of spirit, but accepted that it was a fortunate thing to have a partner that erred on the side of over-generosity than being a miser. I saw how those attitudes could affect relationships, and was glad we had an open and welcoming house to all.

He would always remember birthdays and anniversaries. Even when we didn't have a lot to spend, he would make an occasion of the celebration, and was very romantic. He once cooked and plated up a three-course meal for my birthday worthy of a current Master Chef winner. All under his own steam and from his own imagination.

He treated his mother well, and respected his sisters. If you are looking for how a man will treat you as a woman, this is always a good sign. The difficulties we faced, the values that missed the mark, were exceptions to the rule, and it was only after six years of facing these issues that it became harder to ignore them. They were not there 24 hours of the day, 7 days a week, these would crop up every few months but with enough regularity for me to finally understand they would never be resolved.

He took his responsibilities seriously, and was always striving to be better, the disappointments he felt within himself probably made his "down" cycles worse, which led to further self-esteem issues and fuelling subsequent cycles where he tried to make up for his losses quickly through his gambling episodes.

It was a case of one step forward, two steps back. I just wished and hoped and prayed for the cycles to get further apart or disappear altogether. But without adequate help, diagnosis and medication with therapy, that was probably never going to happen.

Why do all the things I have recounted seem to be such a direct contradiction to a number of other things I have disclosed?

The answer is not simple, and it is not easy to explain. He was, like every other person on this planet, a flawed human being. He was light and dark in varying degrees. He had a beautiful nature that was impacted by some deep deep traumas, and he was a gentle soul who was battling pressures of conformity, sociali-sation, cultural makeup and expectations on him and his life, again like so many of us face.

The subconscious patterns that I have recounted, trying to understand why he didn't want to face them, were the same we all have to deal with to varying degrees. What I am trying to outline is that for John, they were possibly harder for him to face. He may have had an innate fragility that meant looking at the difficult parts of his personality was simply something he could not do.

But in his heart, he was a good man.

In looking back on our issues the only thing that was lacking was acceptance. Acceptance of the struggle, of his issues and of the need to seek, and continue to seek, help. This help could have helped both of us navigate the next few turbulent and increas-ingly painful years of our marriage.

There may have been hope if we could overcome denial.

Chapter Seven

The Decline

My career was taking off, further as I was increasingly sought after as an advisor to some of the major enterprise technology companies both in Australia and throughout Asia Pacific. I had finished my MBA, the culmination of six years studying part time, gaining the top mark in one of my subjects. At the same time I was spending a lot of time travelling throughout Asia Pacific and the US. It seems that the higher my career trajectory soared, the harder I worked at home to keep the disparity from disrupting our lives. It felt like I had two jobs, one as the sought-after advisor, listened to for the sound advice she gave to top C-level executives heading up some pretty major corporations; the other as the deferential spouse willing to put her brain and opinions down more often than not to keep the peace.

Not only that, my increasing travel schedules and added responsibilities of managing a team flung across twelve countries added to the resentment John expressed that I was either living it up while away, or working too hard when at home.

At one point I was asked to relocate to Singapore to be based closer to my team, a solution that seemed like a blessing at the time. But there was only one snag. John couldn't find work in Singapore, at least not the kind that got sponsorship. It was like being offered the world and being reminded that the choices I had made early on in adult life were now making their presence felt in reality.

Something was going to have to give, and once more it was the need for stability and focus on home. I moved on from my high-profile role to take a less demanding job which didn't require international travel and looked forward to some peace and quiet in both work and home life.

John also had a change of heart about his career during this time. Always an excellent salesman, he decided that real estate was the career for him, and we financed his training in the Jenman system, an ethical real estate company that promoted ethics and protecting people. From the outside, it appeared to be the perfect solution for John, who wanted to get ahead in life and career, but in a way that didn't exploit others. However, it did mean we were back to being a single-income household, while John completed training and tried to get a foothold into his newly chosen industry.

I instigated a strict budgeting regime, complete with forecasting cash flows so I could get a warning when things might get tight down the track. It was a work of art, owing to the skills I learned as an analyst with spreadsheets and forecasting tools. It gave me a further sense of control at a time things were clearly not within my sphere of control. Trying to manage a key relationship issue with spreadsheets seems quite funny now looking back on it. But as long as those numbers made sense, my relationship seemed to make sense to me. They became an obsession for me, checking and double checking when costs were incurred, income totted up on the opposite columns, reconciling the gaps with my own little version of board meetings around our kitchen table. I'm sure John got quite suffocated by this sudden micromanagement. His debit cards were also confiscated at this time, something I felt necessary to curb the sudden disap-pearance of our funds. But also the words "domineering bitch" crossed my mind in judgement of myself. How could I emasculate this man so fully? It was a survival tactic.

While John managed to get employment with a local Jenman-certified agency following his training, all was not as it seemed. The flat commission structure on house sales crippled his ability to achieve the financial status he so craved, and forecasting his ability to reach his targets put John back into a depressive state.

At this stage, I was almost giving up on the worn-out speech that hard work and consistency was really the only way to view a career for someone who, by this time, was heading towards his late twenties. Not a trainee in any industry any more.

John watched our friends moving into larger houses, renovating the ones they had, buying nicer cars, having children and going on holidays. It seemed to be a frequent topic of conversation around this time, and my only response was that in all cases our friends had dual incomes in professional careers. Possibly they also were not facing the sporadic gambling losses, something he seemed to forget had an impact!

It was an inconsistent time for John, trying to get ahead but at the same time feeling like he was falling further behind. It would not have mattered so much if the constant comparisons to our social circle were not such a big issue to him, clues of this kept coming up in our discussions all the time. While I tried to assure him that as long as our patch of the world was secure, it didn't matter to me whether we lived in a semi-detached in the western suburbs, or a large house on the North Shore; it was ours all the same. But, it could be any day, week or month that I would return home to find him sitting on the end of our bed, head in his hands. It became the shortcut for "I did it again."

It was like watching a slow train wreck in progress.

* * *

Gamblers Anonymous. Those two words together conjure up all sorts of negative emotions. On the one hand, I was seeking answers, solutions, to the problem. On the other hand, it all seemed so sordid and embarrassing. I had enlisted his parents' support on my own one night, driving solo to sit with them to understand the backstory to this issue. While they could offer me little insight, they did say they would support me in confronting John to seek help, and although I was given a lot of grief for unveiling our problems outside our marriage, together we managed to convince John to attend a meeting.

We walked towards the drab, brown council building. The meetings for Gamblers Anonymous were held in conjunction with Gam-Anon, the support group for spouses of chronic gamblers.

I took comfort in the knowledge that I wasn't alone. But the stories offered by others in that circle were universally depressing. I caught a glimpse of my future in the sagas of the cycle of gambling addictions these partners recounted, their lives always on shaky ground, any grounds gained through savings, property and investments being stripped away through the evils of the pokies, racing forms and TAB. One word that sums up my memories of this night is sordid. I was easily the youngest in the group, and it gave me little hope that my future would be any better looking around at the dour faces of middle-aged men and women who all loved partners who struggled with these inner demons.

I asked all the wrong questions. "How do you stop them?" "How do you get to the bottom of what drives it?" "What strategies can I put in place to minimise the damage?"

It seemed that in many cases, the answer was universally "accept and forgive" and "get out if you don't want to be affected, because they will never change".

Being separated from John's experience, I can offer little insight into his experience of that one meeting we ever went to. However, once again when we debriefed with each other, his whole summary of the night was eerily familiar. "Wow, those people are hard-core gamblers. I am nowhere near that bad."

Translation: "I don't have a problem."

Result: we never went back a second time.

* * *

While privately his world was unstable, with his career in real estate on shaky ground, on the other hand, the face John wanted to present to the world was the man he wanted to be. He got involved in the local Rotary chapter, seeking validation and belonging in a group of professionals whose charter was doing good in the world. But how can you help others when you can't help yourself?

John left the Jenman agent he was employed with, again without notice to myself. We were at my sister's wedding, where I was one of the bridesmaids. He sprung the news on me before the day started, and I can still see some of the strain in my eyes in those photos.

Smiling on the outside, hurting on the inside.

His solution to stress was simply to walk away from it. Don't deal, just quit. Don't face the issue to work out a solution. Minimise.

At this point I was through playing the supportive role. Under no uncertain terms, I instructed him he would be sticking with the real estate sales game, and to find an agency he could work with, one that would allow him to make the commissions he felt entitled to. He did find another short-lived role in a neighbouring suburb, and became quite a successful salesman, winning salesman of the month a few times and getting a bonus incentive of a weekend away.

It seemed to be a time where he was finally on the road to stability. It was run by a team of brothers, where John was the third agent. He did some of his best work there, but ultimately their wheeling dealing ways affected John and he started having doubts about their integrity and ethics.

Once again, I saw storm clouds on the horizon, as the pattern of disillusionment set in.

It's difficult to pinpoint the moment I started pulling away from my marriage. At this point the constant years of treading on eggshells and my inability to trust whether tomorrow would bring the same as yesterday were taking their toll. The stresses and events that within a normal marriage would mean regrouping, communicating and negotiating a suitable outcome for both parties seemed almost impossible for me. I tried, nonetheless, to navigate the ups and downs of the final two years of my marriage with as much optimism and good faith as I could muster.

Something happens to a relationship when trust is lost. My trust in John on a number of essential points had reached an all-time low. There was no infidelity, on either side, but John seemed to almost completely withdraw from me both emotionally and physically. In public he was attentive, loving and as demon-strative as he always was. But at home it was a different matter. Withdrawing into gloomy moods to play video games, watch television or read books were his ways to cope with our relationship becoming more akin to roommates than husband and wife.

I put it down to the firm steps I had taken to ensure our financial stability, and took the blame on my shoulders. I also found it hard to confide in how I was feeling neglected, unloved and unsupported. I didn't want to add to his already seemingly overwhelming emotional burden.

It seemed we were treading water around each other, keeping the peace but not really enjoying a balanced, give-and-take relationship. I would often use the excuse of a late girl's night out with workmates to avoid coming home to a sullen, gloomy mood. John accused me of being too dependent on a glass of wine or two of an evening to relax, with good reason.

John's moods were universally more depressed, not helped by the fact that he had to spend a month recovering from a hospital visit to re-set a formerly broken metatarsal in his foot, from an accident sustained by riding my motorbike too fast to a poker night with my brothers. In his haste, John had missed a car emerging from a side street, and gone flying over the bonnet as he crashed into it, breaking his foot in the process.

He was off work, again, and things were getting dire in our relationship. I recalled a conversation in the car on our way to a friend's house where my inability to express how bad things had become for me was pressing down with the weight of a thousand unsaid remarks, comments just caught on the tip of my tongue in my effort to walk softly around John, afraid of waking Mr Hyde.

"I don't understand why you are not listening to me. What do you want me to do about this? Are you trying to drive me away?" I exploded to an incredulous face. We sat in the car in stone-cold silence for the rest of that trip.

My desire was not about searching for support outside my marriage, my desire burned to fix something irretrievably broken.

* * *

"I can't breathe," were the first words out of my mouth as my sister picked up the phone on her end.

I broke down into tears when she started talking me through the stress I was under.

"I can't do this anymore, I can't go home," I sobbed.

"Where are you?" she replied.

I happened to be sitting on the lowline brick front fence halfway from the local train station and home. My feet had physically refused to carry me close to home, by this time feeling more like a prison than a place of security and stability. It was already dark and cold, winter almost coming to a close. My senses were heightened, like a caged animal ready to spring forth once the gate was up. I could hear the sounds of families getting baths organised, or ready for dinners that I could smell emanating from the brick California bungalows that lined the street I was sitting in. The bus stop was immediately opposite where I sat, and a bus approached, its lights bright in the evening twilight. My arms prickled with goosebumps, uncovered in the cool and slightly moist air. The street lights cast shadows from my form, elongated in the direction I was so unwilling to move in.

"Why don't you go to Mum and Dad's place, can you get there?" My sister's voice broke through my panicked breathing and dull sobs. I felt embarrassed to be openly weeping in plain view of a main thoroughfare, but at the same time I didn't care.

As my breathing calmed a little, my thoughts gathered into what resembled a rational answer to my current predicament.

"No, it's alright, I just needed to let it out. I'll go home."

I did make it home that night, and the next, and the next, but something was broken inside me. I didn't know how to fix it.

* * *

From then on, it seemed everything held meaning in my marriage irretrievably breaking down. A comment here or there, a friend confiding in me about his unhappy relationship, a conversation with John's sister about her divorce and how she was navigating the fallout, a *Simpsons* episode where Homer leaves Marge, a film focusing on an unhappy housewife, and the revenge she wreaked on her unaware husband. I gravitated towards the stories I could relate to, and John grew uncomfortable in what he saw was a trend towards a negative outlook on life within me.

I started to feel isolated, even within my own family and friends. How could they know what I was going through and how could I communicate the depth of my despair and unhappiness to them? John's paranoia was starting to rub off onto me, and I slowly disengaged from people who were once my rocks. I trusted very few people and those who I did trust in became my lifeline to sanity, constantly deferring to them for a reality check about what was real and what was imagined in my outward engagement with John at social occasions. This caused even more paranoia in my relationship, where John saw my confidence in him dwindling, and my reliance on these few people growing. It didn't do anything to improve our situation, but it did keep me grounded.

It felt like I had become a very different person to the one who had met John. I was in survival mode, and barely functional.

Chapter Eight

The Crises

What do you do when you find your marriage stalling owing to lack of trust? You fake it till you think you can make it. I evaluated my options. I had a husband who wanted desperately to prove himself to me, his family and himself that he could succeed in his chosen profession. It was time to really give it everything I had to either support or confront him. I chose the former.

His father had spotted an opportunity and sat us down to discuss it. A small shop front was up for lease in the small shopping village of Sydney's southern suburbs. He and John's mother had recently bought a waterfront property in a neighbouring suburb, so had grown to know the area quite well. The grand plan was to support John's career and, ultimately, have the entire family living near them in a satellite community, something I was never entirely convinced would be suitable for me, but for John seemed like an ideal support network.

John seemed to find a renewed lust for life with this new opportunity. We crunched the numbers and drew up a business plan to go into the real estate game for ourselves. I called our mortgage broker and organised a redraw against the equity I had built up in our home unbeknownst to John, and gave him access to a cash-flow account purely for his business venture. It was like taking a step into uncharted territory, but one I took to demonstrate my faith in him.

The next few months saw our plans come to fruition. John negotiated a three-month lease-free term on the new shop front, and we managed to pull together the entire fit-out, computing environment, marketing materials, website and a potential customer base within three months from ground zero on a shoestring budget. It was a testament to the can-do attitude and the support of our family and friends assisting us getting our new business going, and we opened our doors within a buzz of expectation from the local community that had seen our comings and goings in their shopping centre.

With the benefit of hindsight, it seems from the outside looking in that we had almost made it, it was a question of "just holding on", which made the end all the more shocking and impossible to understand for those not living it.

We'd reached an impasse in our relationship. I wasn't communicating my pain, and John wasn't paying attention to anything other than keeping up appearances. At his best mate's wedding that April, we travelled to the mountain venue in separate vehicles, he in his car, and me on my motorbike in preparation for a group ride I had planned with friends the following day. The separation perfectly summed up our life at that point. We were heading in the same direction, thinking we were on the same page, but in fact we were traversing parallel lives. We had developed very different needs at this point: I needed freedom, ready at a moment's notice to answer the call of the riding group I had grown dependent on to whisk me away from reality; his need was to maintain the appearance a loving couple, on the brink of success.

The wedding video shows us dancing together; our gaze towards each other was loving, but could not depict the inner conflicts we were both facing. It did not show the screaming match I faced the following day as I arrived home from my motorbike trip, unaware I had betrayed John by not arriving before he did, making him look foolish in front of our friend when they arrived to an empty house. I was an unloving, uncaring wife, only concerned with myself. It was an argument I couldn't win, and didn't try to.

At this stage I was confiding in only two friends about the state of my marriage, and getting advice from both. One was married, the other single, both had advice that seemed sane and sound. I was searching for anything that would either help me make it work or help me decide to leave.

While John was researching his prospective client base, I was researching marriage fixes. The first fix was a series of surveys to re-establish stability within our marriage. The surveys seemed breathtakingly simple and based on common sense, and I returned home with hope that we would finally get to the bottom of what both of us needed.

I was not prepared for the storm clouds that passed over John's face as I eagerly explained to him what we were about to do. He was instantly furious, his mouth and eyes twisted in anger and I backed away but was not prepared to back down entirely.

"Can you please give this a go, it seems to be very easy and will help us," I pleaded to his rational side.

Without a word, glowering at me, he took the pencil I was offering and stormed out to the backyard, where we often would sit at the outdoor table for dinner, to read, or relax with each other. He filled out his survey angrily, at one point snapping off the point of his pencil with the pressure he was using.

The fury unleashed within him was troubling for me to witness. Such a simple request, in my eyes, to do something to help our relationship was being met with anger and resistance. At the time I could not see it was more denial; my asking him to face something he clearly did not wish to do was an admission of my feeling that our marriage was failing. He did not like me to express these thoughts to him or to others. That would be admitting the truth.

But you cannot face the truth if you first do not admit there is something to face. The first step towards healing that I myself would later learn.

I surveyed his answers to the survey and compared them with mine. There were clear gaps in all areas, and my heart sank.

It was clear looking at these documents that our values and

emotional needs were further apart than I initially imagined. Attempting to discuss the results was impossible, I had already awoken his anger and it was not the time to face that battle. I would have to put aside my doubts and fears and pick another time to address them.

* * *

Sitting in the cramped office of the marriage counsellor we had been referred to, there were two parts of me present. The first part of me was the one responding to the questions this man was asking me; it was the part of me struggling to articulate what was actually wrong, finding myself glossing over the things that were really bothering me, and playing down the effects they were having. The second part of me was watching myself and John intently, how it was playing out, and how John was reacting, worried he was going to turn into Mr Hyde in front of a third party. He was doing a stellar job of being calm, rational and responding to my issues. I was doing the same for his issues being aired. We were both playing the parts of husband and wife who didn't really need counselling but were here anyway because it seemed like a good idea at the time.

Why are we both acting this way? my alternate ego was yelling at me. *Can't you see you are playing into the denial? What is going on?*

What I fear was going on was my inability as a rescuer, as the enabler in the relationship, to really have my needs heard, especially in the presence of another person.

In one session you cannot unravel the issues of a nine-year relationship, and for me the session resolved nothing, but as we walked back to the car John remarked, "That went well, and I don't think he reckons we need another session."

"You got that from our session?" was my incredulous response.

Once again, I let it go, despairing that we would ever see our relationship with the same lens of inspection or standards. He seemed content to merely look the part of a happy couple, getting validation from this therapist that all was well was enough for him, whereas I desperately wanted to actually be part of a happy couple.

* * *

"What are you watching?" I asked, as I walked into the lounge room from the cold air of the night. The heater made the room warm and inviting. John was sitting on the couch, in a dark mood again, watching the *Simpsons*. Feeling the tension in the air, I sat down to watch, noting that it was the episode where Marge tries to tell Homer she is not happy in their marriage.

"You know, that's exactly how I feel right now," I remarked casually, hoping to lead into another discussion about what could be done about my increasing panic attacks, my further slump into unhappiness and the increasing loneliness I was feeling in our relationship.

"It's always about your needs," snapped John. "I'm doing the best that I can to make you happy and you're never happy. I'm getting dark thoughts again, because nothing I do is working."

This was unfair, I thought. If I never seemed happy it was because I brought up the same issues time and time again. They never were addressed or resolved. So was I supposed to remain silent, and feign happiness, all the while my spirit dimming?

No, I thought, *I will not be silenced for fear of waking Mr Hyde again. This time I will address what is not being discussed.*

"What do you mean dark thoughts," I answered, feeling both concerned and angry that a discussion about how I was continually feeling was being turned again into a discussion on how John didn't want to hear it.

Silence was John's response.

This time my anger overtook my concern for him. I had had enough. I was through having the continual threat of depression and glowering anger, not to mention the implicit threats of self-harm John would make when I tried over and again to explain why I was unhappy, held over my head.

"I am exhausted, John. I cannot continually walk on eggshells around you when you get like this. I don't know what you mean by having dark thoughts, but if you choose to hurt yourself again I would be devastated, but I refuse to guard how I feel anymore."

These words, said calmly and without emotion, were the first time I addressed the problem as I faced it. They would come back to haunt me, but at the time they felt like my saving grace.

* * *

From that point, my courage grew and I started doing things to nurture myself back from my emotional abyss. I felt liberated in my newfound ability to face the truth about my relationship, and I began pulling away. I knew at that point there was nothing more I could do, that if we were facing the end of our marriage that it was simply a matter of time. But I was not ready to face it just yet.

We were still living as husband and wife, but our investment in the relationship was dwindling. John focused on building up his business, looking like it would become very successful as the months passed. Taking heart that his needs were being met, that he was on his way to becoming a very successful independent business owner, and trusted local real estate agent, I organised a week-long break from work with the intention of doing an extended motorbike trip to regional NSW. I included a trip to Parkes and Narrabri for their telescope dishes, an excuse to merely do as much riding as I could using my grandparents' home as my base and an emotionally safe harbour.

On my journey outward, John and some friends came along

as far as Bathurst in their cars, as a farewell party to my adventure. Having lunch at a local pub, I surveyed my husband surrounded by our friends, he seemed to be in good spirits, chatting with the children in our group and generally being his happy self. I thought at the time this was a good sign, he would be okay without me, I believed. He had good friends, and a good support network. There really was no need for me to continue believing I was the only thing he had going for him in life.

After lunch I continued on, shedding many tears beneath my helmet, as I started letting go of my need to be needed. That trip was my spiritual awakening in many ways, as I sought to understand how I contributed to our problem. What we had was not working, I had finally realised, now was my time to take ownership of my part to play in that outcome.

This mode of self-awakening continued on my week-long sojourn away from the stifling presence of being surrounded by my problems, enjoying the ability to take a good look at them from a third-eye observation point and accept what I could and couldn't change. I took back my life in that week, and as I rounded the bends of the backroad coming back from Narrabri, I will always remember the moment the angelic presence of my guide appeared to me as described by meditation practitioners that I had hitherto ignored and never taken seriously.

My senses were all instantly heightened, the movement of the bike became like a chariot to a hidden world, the breeze changed from icy cold to a warm zephyr, time slowed and I could see every blade of grass in the surrounding hillsides. I heard my inner voice saying very calmly and wisely, "You are going to be alright. Stay true to yourself and you shall be set free."

* * *

How does an ending to a marriage happen? Sometimes it's dramatic. Ours wasn't. It was based on a series of innocuous remarks.

"Why can't you be more like your sister?" was one such remark. A couple of weeks had passed since my return from the motorcycle trip. We were sitting in the backyard of my sister and her husband's newly renovated home in a neighbouring suburb, having a delicious dinner that she had prepared, along with a cake she had baked earlier that day.

"I'm not the baking kind of wife, you knew this about me before we got married," I responded, irritated. My sister looked at me, her understanding and compassion for what she could see going on was reflected in her eyes. But of course, she could say nothing.

"I don't know which personality to pick that will please you the most," John said to me in the car on our way home that night. I froze. This was the moment I realised that the marriage was never going to work, not for him and not for me. It was the moment I finally understood what it must be like for John to be married to me, continually trying to switch focus, try something new, something better, do something he hadn't done before to ensure the continuity of a relationship that sustained and supported him, but that he could never be "good enough" for. It had to end, if only for the torture of this kind of existence for John.

The following day, after doing the Saturday reception work for our real estate business, on the way home I told John I wanted a separation. I told him that it was his responsibility this time to ensure his family knew, and that he had all the time he needed until we figured out our next steps.

I also assured him I would help in his real estate business for as long as he needed to continue the stability of it, and that everything would be fair and equitable. I would not make anything difficult. I told him he had the choice to stay at our home and I would leave, or vice versa.

He chose to be the one to leave.

Chapter Nine

The End

That weekend I experienced the most peace I had enjoyed since the beginning of our courtship. I felt light, almost giddy with relief. I couldn't quite believe it had been that easy. But the relief was already tinged with the sadness that my marriage was over. Calling my sister the following morning, I merely had to say "hello" for her to respond "come over now".

I found them gardening, pulling up the old and planning the new. It was an apt metaphor for what I was going through. I said nothing. No explanations were needed as she saw the effects of the previous 24 hours written all over my face. I think she had known for a long time that this was coming, and all she did was hold me tightly. The day was bright, crisp and clear, mirroring my outlook; a fog had been lifted and I could now see a path opening up before me once again.

It's difficult to express the full range of emotions for a passing relationship, let alone one that was complicated by co-dependency. All at once I felt a loss of purpose. While a different path had opened up for me, it also looked very empty and meaningless. If I wasn't saving anyone, then what good was I in the world? I put aside these thoughts and focused on the day, a warm winter day when the only task ahead of me was helping my sister's family replant their garden beds.

I returned home that evening to an empty house, dark and grim. It was the focus of so many memories and once more I was forced to contemplate my situation. I had not heard from John all day, and had let responsibility of his actions fall to him for the first time in our life together.

The following morning I woke up with a sense of foreboding. Unable to face the daily grind, I called work to explain what had happened, and that I would need a few days off to regroup. I knew something was not right, it didn't feel over, and my fear was confirmed when later that afternoon I received a text message from John asking "Can I come home?"

I responded "Did you see the doctor" as he had promised me would be his next action after our separation, and he replied "No, I was too busy".

I sighed a heavy sigh, knowing full well that he was back in the throes of denial. This time I was not going to make everything better. I would be giving him another reality check, and I knew it would get ugly. I steeled my heart and resolve, and pushed aside the fear that rushed up in anticipation of the battle before me, and waited for John to come home.

What mood would he be in, what side of his personality would be present, what approach would he take, all these questions revolved around in my mind as I waited. Finally, sweeping through the front door, I saw John's I-mean-business face approaching me down the hall. Long, purposeful strides, and there was anger in his demeanour.

Thus the battle started. Normally I buckled instantly before John's anger, reacting with soothing diplomacy. This time, I faced him down. While he raged and accused me of everything under the sun, I stood firm. It felt like being in the middle of an angry sea, lashed by waves at every turn, and I imagined myself to be a pillar of iron, with roots deep below the ocean floor.

Nothing he can say will touch me, I thought. *I know the truth and the truth is it's over.*

I clung to that thought and responded with my truth at every turn. I was exhausted, I felt unloved, I felt abandoned and I needed to be on my own to heal. This was my truth and it was all I had left to give him.

He hit walls and paced up and down, yelling and shouting at me. More accusations, more threats, veiled attempts to cower me with physical displays of violence, out of control emotions. A big issue for John seemed to be my lack of desire to have children, "Did you ever want children with me?" I told him this was not the issue. He changed tack, "I knew this was coming ever since you started to confide in other people about our problems."

I replied, "So if you knew there were problems, why didn't you do anything back then to solve them with me?" More anger, and more pacing up and down. This went on for hours.

Still, I was unmoved. I watched him and responded calmly when I could. "I am not trying to hurt you, but it's over. Maybe if you get the help that you need we can rebuild something, but for now I cannot do anything more to help you. You are not helping yourself, you didn't even go to your doctor's appointment. You have not even gone to the dentist appointment I made for you to fix the tooth that's been bothering you. If you can't look after yourself, how can you look after anyone else?"

At that, John's mood went from anger to pitiful. He broke down in tears, and walked to our bedroom. I followed him there, but kept my truth firm in my mind: *I cannot help someone that does not want to help themselves.*

John had laid down on our bed, covering his eyes with his hands. Not seeing? Not wanting to see? Denial? Emotional exhaustion from his display of anger? Not understanding why it was not working as it so often had in the past?

I lay down beside him and hugged him, saying this was not how I envisioned our relationship ending up, that I had done everything I possibly could, but that nothing was working for me. I told him gently that he knew I had done everything possible to resolve things for myself, but that it simply hadn't worked. That he would need to find the strength to heal himself as I would be doing for myself. That in time, maybe one day, we could come back together once we were two strong individuals, but that the time was not now. Not anymore.

He sobbed helplessly, breaking my heart. I did not and never wanted to hurt this man. He sat up in bed, taking off his wedding ring, and placing it on the end of our dressing table, saying, "I said on our wedding that I'd never take this off. But I guess I won't be needing it anymore."

Those words chilled me, but still I remained firm to my truth, "I wish you didn't feel the need to do or say that, but know that it will be here, just in case."

He turned to look at me, and I could clearly see the pain in his eyes. "I wish this place were bigger so that we could live together but separately." How could the agony in my heart get any worse?

"John," I said gently, my heart breaking at his need of me. "That is not our answer."

One more gut-wrenching sob and he tore himself off the bed, and to the front door. I got up as he opened it, and called after him as he ran to the car. "John! Where are you going now? Does your family know?"

He didn't answer. I watched as he got in the car, and looked over at me standing in the doorway. The car's interior light showed his face crumple once more in pain, the most agonised I had ever seen him. Like an entirely different person. One last glance at me, and he sped off into the night.

* * *

"Mum, I can't find John anywhere, he's not answering his phone or text messages. I've looked at our credit-card transactions and he hasn't stayed anywhere last night."

"What are you going to do?"

"Should I report him as a missing person? I'm scared, Mum, what if he comes back?"

"Do you think he will hurt you?"

"I just don't know. I have never felt this scared before, so maybe. I just don't know."

"You'd better come to our place then."

"No, if he comes back here, I want to be here."

"You should tell his family."

"Okay."

* * *

The police were clearly not taking me seriously. Or at least, the cocky younger one who was wandering through my lounge room, looking at my things, was displaying body language that clearly read "I haven't got time for hysterical chicks" while the older sergeant who was obviously in charge was entertaining my story with extreme politeness.

"He's been missing since when, you say? Last night?"

"Yes."

"Has he done this sort of thing before?"

"Well no, but...."

"What leads you believe he has come to harm, or may be a danger to himself?"

How do you explain nine years of harm and denial, precipitated with an attempted suicide? I tried my best to outline the situation, but told in ten minutes, my story did seem rather implausible and weak.

Still, they took my details and I had spoken with his father and mother that morning, putting them on the alert as well. His father had sounded fairly positive, saying, "Don't worry, he will come around, I'm sure."

The following morning, his mother called to see whether I had any word. No, I said. "This is making me feel nervous," she said, "it's bringing back memories and feelings I had from a long time ago."

She didn't need to elaborate, I knew what she meant.

* * *

I stripped the bed clothes, smelling his scent on them as I put them in the washing machine. It was another crisp, clear winter's day, the last day of winter in fact, Wednesday 31st of August, 2005.

The warm sun dried the linen in record time, and I remade the bed, lying down in it and enjoying the freshness. I checked how I was feeling, and suddenly realised I couldn't feel him anymore. When you live with someone for that length of time there is an energetic bond that ties you together. I couldn't feel that bond anymore. I think that was the moment I knew.

The doorbell rang.

When you see police at your door, looking serious, you know what is about to come. Still, I acted normal. I felt normal. I asked them in. It was the same policemen that took my statement the previous day. I observed without emotion how embarrassed the younger one looked. I knew why.

They followed me down the narrow hallway of my semi-detached house.

I sat down in the corner chair. They remained standing. I waited for the words to come.

"I'm very sorry to inform you that your husband was found in his car in a side street off the Bells Line Road this morning. He has passed away."

In the distance of my mind, I heard a primal scream. My head was throbbing, and my senses muted as though hearing sounds while underwater. As the sounds cleared, I realised the sound was coming from me.

I can't remember how I got to be sitting on the edge of my bed, with the phone in my hands, sobbing. But that's where my memory kicks back in. The phone was in my hands, I must have dialled my mother's number somehow and all I could do in between my loud cries, was to force out, "He's gone, Mum, he's gone..."

I dropped the phone after I heard her say, "I will be there

right away, darling."

The police asked whether they could wait with me, I simply nodded and kept sobbing. I kept sobbing until my mother arrived and held me in her arms, nothing could ever feel right again, I thought. Nothing.

There is no description for the pain you feel when someone takes their life. No words. Just a big black hole of despair, emptiness, and horror. The horror of the truth that they have overcome man's strongest instinct to stay alive and brought about their own end to life, is what you feel. It comes in waves of nausea, after the initial shock, and keeps hitting you, and hitting you, over and over again.

Why?

Why?

Why?

* * *

All of a sudden, that night my little house became the focal point for everyone to gather. I felt overwhelmed with the love and support but at the same time I was overwhelmed by my emotions and my hold on reality was tenuous. After crying for hours, until my tears literally ran dry, I started laughing and chatting with each new person who came to pay their respects. After a few hours I appeared to be completely normal, laughing and talking normally, but in reality I had gone into shock.

We swapped stories about John's life, and I was so grateful for all the laughter and shared moments we had of his life. That night felt like a celebration for his amazing nature, wonderful larger-than-life personality, his affection for everyone, and his sense of humour. We focused on all the good things to ward off the horror. The descent of his spirit, his trauma, and his suppressed and denied demons. Those were not up for discussion that night.

Much later, after reading everything I could get my hands on about grieving and suicide, a common theme became apparent. Grieving for a suicide has a lot more denial involved, given the feelings of guilt and self-recrimination that are tied up in losing someone in such a sudden and unexpected way. Even though I was telling everyone around me I had seen it coming, I really hadn't accepted that it could ever happen. In some part of me, it hadn't actually happened, and that's the way I felt for a very long time. I was struggling with the truth of it, and couldn't process it, therefore, it could not have happened.

Recounting stories about what people had been doing when they heard of his demise became par for the course, and almost comforting, as if reinforcing the boundaries of reality. It's easy to give into denial, and so the endless storytelling became a way to get a grip on reality once more.

Parts of my life for the next few weeks and months were so dreamlike that looking back now and recounting what I went through is like dictating someone else's storyline. Each fresh horror cemented in my mind that, *This is not real, it can't be real, such things just don't happen to normal people.* And I desperately wanted to cling to the vision that I was normal, or what kind of life could I ever possibly look forward to ever again?

The police asked for a family member to identify John. I was not in any state to do so, and the task fell to my brother and brother-in-law. The most loving thing my brother-in-law could ever do for me was done this night, when he described the moment they pulled the sheet from him, saying, "He looked like he was sleeping." I imagined him asleep, peaceful, which was what I desperately wanted for him. To be at peace at last.

The funeral was another dream. I recall very little, other than clinging onto my sister, laughing hysterically inside the church after the funeral directors had brought the casket in, reading out my eulogy, watching the casket descend into the ground from afar, and hearing the thuds from the clumps of dirt that we each dropped onto his casket.

It just did not seem real. It was all a joke.

The following weeks were also like another world. I became overly bubbly, bright, trying to overcompensate for others' pain. If I could just fix everyone else, then eventually I would be fine. I had to recount the events leading up to his disappearance for his family. Understandably, questions were asked and I did my best to give the answers. But at this point nobody could answer the ultimate question: Why?

Not even me.

The police came once more to ask for a statement of events leading up to John's death. They also wanted to understand the nature of our relationship. Spending three hours at a police station trying to describe my relationship was possibly the most surreal experience I went through during this time. The officer was very understanding and started confiding in me about his relationship, and I once more found myself being the shoulder for someone else's relationship woes, a laughable situation given the circumstances! But, as always, I took the chance to focus on someone else rather than what I was going through at the time. A theme that would recur many times through the following years of recovery whenever my pain became too much to examine.

The guilt I felt at being the catalyst for him deciding to take his own life was undeniable, and my self-worth plummeted along with my mental capacity for coping with even the smallest tasks. On my own now, by choice yet somehow also not by choice, the task of getting on with life now seemed insurmountable.

Sleep was elusive, so I turned to drinking heavily to knock myself out at night. Waking up groggy and already mentally drained from denying my grief, I struggled through the tasks of winding up his business affairs, preparing to return to work and trying to figure out what my next steps should be.

My life suddenly lost all colour, all meaning, and literal darkness now shrouds all memories of those first few months.

Chapter Ten

The Aftermath

As people gathered around me over the next few weeks and months, descending in their own reaction to grief and shock at the news, I went into my own kind of denial. I was fine, absolutely fine, I assured everyone. I had had nine years to come to terms with this outcome, and how was everyone else going? Are you okay? How about you? Do you need a hug, or a chat, or to express your feelings about what has just happened?

I went into uber-coping mode, a switch had gone on in a deep part of my psyche that I didn't know existed, and I blanked my own feelings out and pushed my needs so far down that I became everyone else's tower of strength, on and off, for the next few months.

Of course, I was not being strong, and it was incredibly naive of me to think I could escape my grief forever. But that became my battleground, and I squared off with grief, unable to look it directly in the eyes, and danced the dance of denial for a very long time.

For a while I heard comments like "She will be okay, she's strong" and despaired inwardly. I was not strong, I was not coping. But I lacked the ability to communicate this message; my emotional tools were all geared towards helping others, not myself.

My journal entry from 30th September, 2005 describes my inner turmoil:

I am sitting in the backyard crying. I went to bed earlier, about midnight, but I can't stop my thoughts. Thoughts like "I want to die". And why it feels like everyone is failing me, even though I think I've been asking and asking and asking for help. I keep telling people I am incapable of doing anything.

I've been so used to being capable, being able to pick up the pieces, and I'm so afraid that this time I will not be able to do it. Is this the time I have a complete breakdown? I look so normal on the outside and yet inside I am dying. I can feel my heart hardening towards everyone, and I'm scared that it will be too late to stop it and I will end up alone, with no friends or family because I will have alienated everyone. I wish I could put a stop to this relentless pain that just won't go away.

I've never needed rescuing in my life before, but right now I could use some pretty drastic rescuing.

Why can't I stop sobbing?

Make the pain go away.

Make the pain go away.

Make the pain go away.

Make the pain go away.

Make the pain go away.

By this time, my grief was in full swing, whether I admitted it or not. I bounced from denial to anger to bargaining to sadness and despair right back to denial again. It was a circular loop on a train going nowhere. I was good at beating myself up for mistakes I made, and even those mistakes that others made during this time, but I shouldered them all, as the well-trodden co-dependent pattern within me dictated.

I broke every rule in the grief handbook that is supposed to help you get through it relatively sane and intact. I drank copious amounts of wine to medicate the pain. I let my health go, stopped exercising, took up chain smoking, put on weight and ate badly. I pushed people away, then clung desperately to them, in alternate measures. I acted like a crazy person while trying desperately to pretend I was normal.

I threw myself into online dating, trying to recapture what I had lost so very recently, in order to go on with life as though it had not been interrupted by this huge event that I was unwilling to disclose to anyone. I conducted those dates and affairs extremely badly. Unsurprising, given I had never dated much in the first place before John, and hadn't the faintest sense of what was normal, and given my almost negligible self-esteem, I only attracted the most hodgepodge group of losers and abusers that simply reinforced my view that my life would only ever hold more pain, grief and dysfunction.

And rock bottom had yet to come!

The entire year of 2006 became about finding love to deny the pain of loss. Another journal entry from the first of March, 2006 pinpoints a critical point with a failed relationship attempt:

I am being held back by all these messy emotions. I was diagnosed a few weeks ago with atypical depression and PTSD. It was a low point to think I actually need medication to deal (sic). Last week I was sent a poem which sent me off the rails again. My reaction was so visceral it freaked me out. Anger washed over me to think my emotions can still be so easily manipulated and wrung out again.

Refusing to take the medication that was prescribed to me, I fell further and further into spirals of depression throughout 2006. During this time, I also bought a new place to live as I couldn't bear living in "our" house any longer than necessary. A bright new trendy loft apartment in the inner city became a little oasis for my depression in the latter half of the year, but I still held onto the house, unable to part with it just yet.

There were also big changes to come within the job that I loved, shaking my security once again, with a rival company buying us out, with the ensuing departure of key staff (and friends) as well as a culture change almost overnight. More change is simply not possible to cope with when you are already dealing with unresolved grief and stress. This became a tipping point.

Self-hatred becomes ingrained and very difficult to turn around, and I had to reach rock bottom before I realised this. During the year it had felt like my anchor was ripped from its mooring, and I let myself go on a pendulum swing of emotions, hoping that by the time it stopped I would be where I needed to be to finally start my life anew.

What precipitated the end of my struggle with denial was a friendship being terminated with the instructions "don't contact me again". It seemed to be the final paragraph to my tale of loss and self-loathing, reinforcing to my mind that indeed I was nothing and would never amount to being anything for anyone ever again.

I hadn't slept for a week at this point, and in my grief decided the best way through the pain would be to end it.

I took a bottle of sleeping tablets and swigged what was left of the alcohol I had lying around the kitchen, went upstairs to my bedroom, lay down on my bed and waited for sleep to come, knowing I may never wake up again. I felt relief at last, thinking the pain would be over, finally.

I felt my breathing slow down, and my heart seemed to thump less regularly, but I didn't mind the sensation, it was soothing, like a slowing down lullaby, lulling you off to sleep.

But with suicide, you're not simply ending your pain, you're giving it to someone else.

That someone else would be my family, the people who loved and supported me unconditionally throughout everything I had been through. I suddenly thought of what my actions would do to them, and how they would feel. I could not do this to them, they didn't deserve this pain.

It was an effort, but I roused myself and stumbled into my bathroom, next to the bedroom in the upstairs loft. I then managed to get downstairs and outside where I hailed a taxi that happened to be passing that very moment, groggily mumbling, "St Vincent's Hospital please."

I sat in a stretcher in the emergency department, having had my stomach cleared, but no beds were available to me. So I called my best friend to keep me awake as I had been instructed by the nursing staff, chatting about things completely unrelated to my surroundings.

No one knew.

I had decided that was the moment I would face it and get better, come what may. I didn't know whether I would ever feel normal again, but I was going to make it my life's mission to try. It was an act of blind faith, this moment. I can't say I felt any better, I would not feel better for a very long time, but that was the turning point and decision to get real with myself and with life.

Denial would never be an option again.

Chapter Eleven

Back to Me

The first step towards healing is recognising you have a problem. If I hadn't by now recognised that I had a problem, my life was certainly giving me more warnings that would only get stronger and more dramatic if I didn't heed them. I knew, as I pondered my way forward over the next few weeks, that something had to change. The only problem was I had no idea what that was or what I needed to do in order to change it.

The only thing I was sure of, as the following journal entry describes, was the denial and deception.

8th January, 2007

I need to take responsibility. I have reached clarity of myself now, of my actions. This unconditional love that I have been writing about? I didn't show it. If I judge myself on my actions and behaviour, rather than my words, it reveals a very ugly side of my character.

If I also look at the way I behave with my family and friends, it also reveals a pattern of behaviour. I accept responsibility for that and accept that I can change it to avoid repeating the same mistakes again.

How do I change this? By restoring my integrity.

Integrity of thoughts: I will, with intention, think only pure thoughts of others.

Integrity of word: I will keep my counsel, only speak well of others, make promises I can keep and be honest in all expressions of intent. I will speak well of myself.

Integrity of actions: I will follow through on my word and do the things I promise to do. I will behave in a calm manner and treat others as I would like to be treated.

When I seek advice and help it will be with good intentions.

> *When I offer help and advice and behave generously it will be with the intent of not seeking favours in return.*
> *When I thank someone it will be with the intent of expressing gratitude for that action, and not because I hope for it to continue.*
> *I will be true to myself and believe in myself.*
> *Integrity. Respect. Humility. Self-belief. Kindness.*

I didn't realise it then, but I was scripting the goals I would aspire to for the rest of my life and the standard I wished to hold myself to. I still had no idea how to do it. But I had faith that once I set my intention, and remained vigilant, a sign would be shown to me.

But what about this behaviour I thought I displayed? Where did that come from? By this time I felt I had been putting on an Oscar award-winning performance for most of my life. As the eldest child in a family of four children, I was a typical "first child", stressed and anxious, always trying to play the family hero and taking the weight of the world on my shoulders. Outwardly I appeared happy, charismatic and successful but inwardly I felt the ever-present knife of anxiety, and I had suppressed feelings of bitterness and resentment most of my life.

Because I had learned to keep my feelings buried as a child, I continued to deny and suppress negative feelings as an adult, giving me a warped perspective on conflict, rejection and issue-solving. I often confused pity with love, tending to love those I thought I could rescue. As long as I wasn't trying to fix me, it was okay.

I moved forward in a dysfunctional and wounded adulthood using alcohol or food, overachievement, workaholism and co-dependent relationships to numb my pain. I ran as far away from my home, my family and myself as I could, to escape from the torture of being me but there was never really a place far away enough to run.

I saw the clarity finally, that I was constantly putting tiny Band-Aids on what turned out to be a fatal wound, left unchecked and untreated for far too long. Having been a habit for so long, I felt oddly comfortable nailed to the cross and bleeding.

It was time to free myself from all of these patterns of behaviour, thoughts, and bring myself back to self-love. It would be a journey that spanned more than five years, and continues to this day. But at the beginning it took a single step, and the belief that I would keep taking a step and then another, and another, and another, until I found myself in a place of peace and balance.

The first major signpost that I was pointed in the right direction came two weeks after that journal entry. An old and inactive online dating profile sprang back into life with a message sent to me by someone who resonated with me so strongly I was compelled to respond.

My friendship with Raphael began with, what can only be described as a spark of recognition between two souls that knew they were destined to help each other in the purest sense. The friendship was never fated to be a partnership in the usual sense of the word, but one of spiritual warriors meeting at the beginning of a journey of self-discovery.

Make no mistake, these kinds of friendships are no happy-ever-after tales. They are not easy. They are difficult in the way they challenge you and shake you up in ways you sometimes wish not to have to go through. But in the end, they leave you better people and more accepting of what you needed to learn.

I was constantly pushing the boundaries in our friendship, believing connection to equal love. I was continually disappointed to learn this was never going the way I wanted it to. It was my first lesson in learning to let go of my idea of what unconditional love felt, looked and acted like. It was the ultimate practical test of my ability to just accept, go with the flow, and allow love into my life in forms other than romantic love. At the time, I chose to see it as not being worthy of love. Looking back, my worthiness of love was being demonstrated to me through the universe giving me the chance to be loved by someone with no other designs on me other than mutual help through our trials and life lessons.

During my friendship with Raphael I was introduced to the concept of spiritual development. He taught me that being "self-ish" during this time of healing when we have to restock our resources and heal past wounds, was as important as being self-less at other times when we have enough to give others. Challenging my long-held belief that I would be a bad person if I focused only on myself, Raphael taught me that being purely "self-less" could be damaging to one's spirit, and that focusing on self was actually the highest pursuit of spiritual development.

Over the next three years I studied with a spiritual teacher who taught guided meditation founded in Buddhist principles. I was introduced to a holistic approach to spiritual development. The practice taught me to connect to myself in a deeper way on a spiritual plane, and gave me the tools to see where obstacles presented themselves, and how to dissolve them with unconditional love.

The principles of the meditation practice I followed were based on the following key tenets:

1. We are all spiritual beings having a physical experience.
2. The only truth is unconditional love, the source of that unconditional love comes from the Creator.
3. All of our suffering, our pain, darkness, and struggles are derived from our ego.
4. We are all here for a reason, to learn the lessons we decided to learn pre-birth, to resolve karma and reach the next level of consciousness.
5. Even after learning all that we can learn about spiritual development, we still have to live in the real world.

One can spend a lifetime learning the intricacies of all these principles, and there are a set of Buddhist teachings that will go further than this, but I only explored those that helped me reach my own understanding of life, and how I got meaning back into mine.

It was not a fun time, though, and it was a lot of hard work. I asked many questions and questioned the answers I got, I spent a lot of time and energy blaming myself for where I was in life, trying to find absolution and forgiveness and seeking signs that I was cured. I recall now with a laugh the many times my teacher would ask after a meditation what I had seen and how I interpreted the messages by identifying feelings. I would always begin "I think...." he would immediately respond "No, don't think, what did it feel like?" I often simply could not answer him. It was the first of many signs that I was not connected to my emotions or emotional body at all. I could not interpret how I felt.

What I did feel was the need to get back to normality instantly. Now that I had made the decision to be better, I wanted to be better right away, and not have to wait a moment more for life to begin anew. I spent many sessions in tears wondering, *When will I get there? When does this end and I can say I am better?* I was driven by impatience, and a desire to have a normal life immediately.

And what was a normal life, according to my ego? To love and be loved again, of course. To get the chance to "do it right" this time, and not throw it all away like I felt I had done. This outlook was the reason my path was long and hard to reach the understanding that my life would never be the same again, and that acceptance of that, and compassion towards myself were going to be the only tools I would need to feel whole again.

Learning patience for an impatient person is one of the hardest lessons in life. And spiritual development is only one aspect in the mind-body-spirit trinity of health.

My mental health had been suffering along with my spirit. Not to mention my body was locked from both physical and emotional pain.

The next signpost in my search for balance came when I sought treatment for the shallow breathing I found restricting both my movement and my wellbeing. At first I thought it was the result of inflamed asthma, something I had suffered from since childhood. I had heard that the Buteyko breathing technique was the best way to free oneself from medicated asthma, so I looked for a practitioner and started treatment sessions.

One session, I found myself lying on the floor with cushions all around me, to help my body learn the optimal sleeping position for opening my lungs, and I suddenly found myself openly weeping and unable to stop. I was incredibly embarrassed, but my teacher was instantly soothing and calmed me back to the point of talking about what had happened.

I couldn't explain what had happened, I was oblivious to my feelings at this point, all I felt was overwhelming sadness when put into the sleeping position, something that prevented me from getting a good night's sleep, and I avoided bedtime until I couldn't stay awake any longer on the couch.

Seeing this was out of her area of expertise, she recommended I see a kinesiologist who specialised in releasing the emotional stress and trauma locked in my body, something that I had only heard of in reference to sporting injuries, never to emotional injuries. But again, my whole body tingled, and I knew this was a sign to take seriously.

* * *

My first experience with kinesiology was intense and liberating. I walked into the well-appointed Californian bungalow on Sydney's lower North Shore to be greeted by a pleasant yet no-nonsense woman who was to open the door to a new world of self-discovery.

It is interesting to note, after the fact, the signposts and warnings that are being shown to you every day, that you later discover you should not have ignored. I had heard of this woman many times a few years before, from colleagues at the company I worked for when John passed away. While I was intrigued enough to ask what she did and how kinesiology worked, and why it was spoken of in such a reverent way by people I admired and respected, I never took up the urgings to book an appointment.

Now, here I was, nervously anticipating what lay in store for me on the other side. She took me into the front room, and I lay down on the massage table, while she asked a few questions about why I was there, how I was feeling and what I wanted to get out of the day's session.

I briefly explained the series of events that led up to my visit, the breakdown I had with my Buteyko breathing teacher, and a very very short version of what had happened in my life in the previous few years. I explained that I had trouble breathing when walking up even slight slopes, my body felt stiff and locked all the time, and I would like to get some relief from the pain. All the while I spoke, she used my arm like a lever, and when it stayed strong she said I was "congruent with what you are saying" and when it flopped down to the table, she told me "your body doesn't agree with you".

I was fascinated.

She got to work immediately, starting at the top of my body and working her way down, her fingers seemed to immediately encounter knots of pain at each and every point that she worked on over the next two hours. I tried to bear the pain as much as I could, while she talked through the points on my body she was finding, the meaning behind each of them, and the typical emotional responses they bring up in us. Her voice and words kept me from leaping off the table, saying "enough" and walking out the door, and I understood that we were releasing almost at a DNA level the lifetime of emotions and tension that I had kept locked in my body.

That session was a rollercoaster ride of pain, tears, yet the absolute assurance that I was releasing something that I didn't need to carry within me anymore. My kinesiologist's firm yet caring touch, along with her ability to connect the dots for what I was experiencing with what I had experienced in my past, sometimes bringing up details I had not discussed and she could not have known from the brief explanation I had given, was opening up the first gateway to my understanding that my body itself was an emotional weathervane that I had been ignoring my entire life. The intuitive nudges, the warning bells, the signs that I was not doing what was best for me, were being awakened with a jolt, and old energy streams within me that had lain dormant were being urged to break through the barriers blocking them, and start moving again.

During later sessions, she explained to me she had spent as much time as was necessary to open up every single energy channel within my body, all blocked up to that morning. She could not let me leave without doing this, she explained later, or the chances of me coming back to finish the task were next to zero.

She possessed an amazing ability to read me better than I could read myself, all through signs my body gave her. I wanted to know more. During the next few sessions I asked her questions about what she was doing, how she came to do what she was doing, and what was the best way for someone like me to learn more.

* * *

There was another aspect to my life that was developing in parallel with the spiritual healing and physical wellbeing I was focusing on. The fun side of life that I had been disconnected to for such a long time was in much need of a boost. Again, not consciously aware of the path I was on, but trusting my instincts about what felt right for me, I began exploring the side of myself that had been locked away while looking after someone else, my love of performance and music.

Feeling like I had nothing to lose, considering I already felt I'd lost everything, I put myself forward in ways I never did in the past. I introduced myself to musicians who struck a chord with me, I followed them to their gigs, meeting new people and discovering more amazing bands, and so the knock-on effect continued.

One of my very dear friends recently described her first encounter with me during this period. "I had to make a decision whether to consciously follow up on your offer of friendship, or whether to let it go," she recalled. "You seemed so eager, like a puppy discovering a new playmate, it was overwhelming. But in the end, there was something about you that was so honest that I stayed in touch."

We both are very grateful that she did. I am sure there were others during this time that felt this way, and who could blame them? I was like a born-again anything, rediscovering a zest for life, even when at times I didn't feel it, the zealousness of my passion to treat every day like a blessing and my determination to make my life something better than it had been, could have been very off-putting to some, and intriguing to others. Those who have stayed the distance have become some of the most wonderful, warm, and amazing friends that I could have believed myself having.

This is the outcome of trusting in your intentions. Even when it feels like you are treading water, as I did so many times during these years, when you look back on how it all unfolds you realise that the universe was always protecting you, there to give you a sign or a warning about people, events and circumstances. And it inspires you to believe and trust some more.

My love of performance and desire to break free of my own

self-doubt led me to take a huge leap of faith in 2008. I signed up to learn Theatresports improvisation. Terrified that I would make an absolute idiot of myself, I had flashbacks to my university days when I first tried my hand at this exhilarating artform. Back then, however, my experience was soured by a teacher that seemed more intent on pointing out my failures than explaining how to let go of the fear and say "yes, and..."

Thank goodness I found a better set of teachers this time. By the time I had completed both levels of the workshops, the little troupe that had formed quite a close bond were told we would be putting together a graduation performance. The prospect of performing in front of an audience, made up of family and friends of course, was terrifying. But the little voice inside my head just kept saying, "It's only a game, just have fun".

I considered it a very positive sign when I was walking to the venue of our graduation night performance, and encountered one of my friends from the troupe. He was one of the most laidback guys I had ever met, and his absolute confidence and belief that we should just "have fun" was inspiring to me before the show.

Our troupe went on to put on a fantastic show, and I won "Moment of the Match", which was then replayed in slow motion at the end of the show. It was the biggest high I had experienced, and I signed myself up to continue performing in Scared Scriptless, at the time the longest running comedy show in Sydney.

My social life seemed to be getting a kick-start again. At the same time I was working on myself, I was managing to make new friends and feel valued in a social sense again.

* * *

The answer to the ultimate question, what is the meaning of my life, has always been an obsession for me. Using the humorous answer "42" from Douglas Adam's *Hitchhikers Guide to the Galaxy* has been a knowing nod to the fact that I will probably never get a clear answer, or at least one that satisfies my need to know "everything". But it is my quest, nonetheless.

When I started studying my Certificate IV in kinesiology in 2009, I believed I had finally found the answer to "Why am I here?" The year began promisingly enough, I was enrolled in a course, I was employed in a role that spanned the financial and technology world, and I felt like things were on the right path for the time being.

How wrong I was. Two months into my course I found myself let go from my job owing to the financial downturn. It was a moment that could have sent me back off the rails, disappointed with life handing me more obstacles and turning my back on what I had believed my path to be.

I sat in the boardroom having heard I was being "let go", and smiled at my boss who so clearly didn't want to be giving me this news. I knew, in that moment, with absolute conviction, that everything was going to be alright. I didn't know how, but I knew this was a test. I just smiled and said I didn't need to take a day to adjust, and that I would be happy to work out my notice.

As it turned out, I was offered a fantastic role working with a philanthropy division of a large multinational company four days later via contacts I had made earlier in my career. It was to be the beginning of another very happy working environment, and one that opened my eyes to another world of possibilities.

Again, I found the trust and faith to believe that things will work out the way they are supposed to. My old anxiety and depression were already being given the heave-ho through the work I had done to date. Once I let go of my fear, expectations and aversion to change, the world opened up to me in ways I thought wasn't possible.

A second test came that year when the kinesiology course I had enrolled in turned out to be another challenge. It made me question the path I was taking, but once again I found within myself the strength and insight to see that the path was correct, but the course I had chosen may not be ideal. Swiftly and decisively I made the adjustments necessary to continue my education in this inspirational modality in surroundings that were more conducive to my needs. It was another practical test in meeting my own needs, and not those of others, and I had passed with flying colours, and found myself increasingly happy that year and finishing my studies by gaining three certifications in kinesiology.

Things settled down again for a while, as I forged ahead in all areas – in my career, in healing myself and others through kinesiology, and having fun with music and improvisation.

* * *

But what of romance?

It has become my understanding that the very thing we attach to causes the most pain. And my attachment to needing to love and be loved in a romantic sense has caused the most setbacks on my path. During the entire six years following John's death, I kept up the assumption that I would know I had made it out of the woods by the fact that I would be chosen again by someone special. Someone who was special to me. It would be easy, there would be no dramas, it would be the same as when I had met John for the first time, we would just recognise each other.

Sadly, this assumption has meant making a lot of mistakes in this area. Each setback has rattled my self-confidence and belief that I am worthy of love. Each time I seek to understand where things went wrong. Each time I thought I had messed up.

When a cycle of relationship patterns keep coming back to teach you lessons you refuse to learn the first time around, it is time to wake up and notice. A recurring pattern that kept testing my integrity and perspective kept happening throughout the entire time I spent working on myself. The final time I made space in my life for the pattern to play out, I made the conscious decision to really look at what was going on, to resolve what needed resolution, and to trust and let go of the attachments I had previously kept once a relationship had dissolved.

What I noticed was that my need to be needed was stronger than my need to have equality in my partnerships. It was the first time this was shown to me so clearly that I immediately stopped what I was doing, and let go of the need. The people who were meant to be in my life stayed. Those who were not meant to be there, those who could not take responsibility for their own paths of healing, went away. It all became crystal clear.

I don't have to be anyone's saviour to feel loved. I am just meant to be, and believe that good things are coming my way. And that is more than enough.

Epilogue

Two years after this book was written, and exactly one year before her 40th birthday, Natasha was on the cusp of a new job that was to give her newfound independence as well as the recognition for 20 years of hard work building a career in both marketing and journalism. Finally reaching the point where she was at peace with her life, she looked back on the hard work taken to reach this peak, thinking, *I'm okay. I'm finally okay with everything.*

The following day she went to shut down her old online dating profiles, feeling perfectly content to just be on her own indefinitely. She noticed a new message, and out of curiosity read it. The message was simple, yet something compelled her to respond.

Through that exchange and many more than followed, she met and fell in love with her current partner, who she has been with since that day. She looks back on the words within this book, and her experience with John, with fondness and a recognition that sometimes we must go through trials to learn who we are really capable of, and how much love we are able to give.

~The End~

About the Author

Sydneysider Natasha David explored many avenues of assistance to overcome the debilitating depression and anxiety she experienced following her husband's sudden death. Meditation, the Buteyko breathing technique and kinesiology were some of the tools she explored in her recovery from grief and heartbreak. The latter proved so successful in enabling her to release the stress and internalised emotions from the trauma of losing her husband that she became a certified kinesiology practitioner.

Now 42, she advocates meditation as a method to calm the distracting chatter that occurs in our heads during times of stress or trauma, known as "monkey mind" in Buddhist teachings.

The cumulative result of these practices delivered Natasha to the point where she could write about her painful and difficult story with detachment and compassion. She believes love and empathy can overcome any trauma and can help bring understanding for those in pain and suffering.

About Marrying Bipolar

On the last day of winter, John committed suicide in his car on a lonely side road of the Blue Mountains to the west of Sydney, Australia. He was six months shy of his 30th birthday. It was the culmination of nine years of struggle for John and his wife, as he battled undiagnosed mental illness, a gambling addiction, and an earlier suicide attempt. Despite his wife's love and attempts to understand his condition, in the end nothing could save John from his demons.

Tragically, John's story could be anybody's story. In Australia, around 2,100 people commit suicide every year; up to 12% of people affected by mental illness take their own lives, and suicide is the main cause of premature death among people with mental illness. But the effects of suicide are even more far-reaching. Its impact on those left behind is frequently devastating and lifelong.

Author Natasha David knows this firsthand. *Marrying Bipolar* is the account of a wife's struggle to understand the events in her husband's life that would eventually lead to their marriage breakdown and his untimely death.

Natasha's experience watching her husband struggle with the complexity of mental illness, has led her to understand the deadly role denial has to play, for both sufferer and partners. In the process, the author addresses her own search of ways to address denial of the darkness that resides in all of us, and the compassion needed to heal and rebuild lives after enduring.

Soul Rocks is a fresh list that takes the search for soul and spirit mainstream. Chick-lit, young adult, cult, fashionable fiction & non-fiction with a fierce twist.